Traction and Orthopaedic Appliances

Traction and Orthopaedic Appliances

by

JOHN D. M. STEWART

M.A. (Cantab.), F.R.C.S. (England)

Consultant Orthopaedic Surgeon
Chichester & Graylingwell, and Worthing,
Southlands & District Groups of Hospitals

(formerly Lecturer in Orthopaedics,
Institute of Orthopaedics, Royal National
Orthopaedic Hospital, London)

CHURCHILL LIVINGSTONE
Edinburgh London and New York 1975

CHURCHILL LIVINGSTONE

Medical Division of Longman Group Limited
Distributed in the United States of America by
Longman Inc., New York and by associated
companies, branches and representatives throughout
the world.

First published 1975

ISBN O 443 01196 6

Library of Congress Catalog Card Number 74-80738

Filmset on 'Monophoto' 600 by
Fyldetype Limited, Kirkham, PR4 3BJ, England

649
orthopaedics

Printed in Great Britain.

Preface

This book is written primarily for the use of orthopaedic house surgeons and junior registrars, and of the nursing and physiotherapy staff of accident and orthopaedic wards.

Many of the procedures and appliances described here are in common usage. The details, however, of how to carry out these procedures, their contraindications and complications, and how to check the various appliances, are not available in the standard textbooks. This book is intended to rectify this omission and to be a practical source of instruction in these matters.

I wish to thank the many people who have assisted me in the preparation of this book, in particular Mr W. H. Tuck without whose considerable guidance, the chapters on Spinal Supports, Lower Limb Bracing and Footwear would have been incomplete; Dr J. D. G. Troup for his help with the section on the biomechanics of the spine; Mr F. G. St.C. Strange and Mr G. R. Fisk who have kindly helped me in the description of their methods of applying traction to the lower limb; and to the staff of the Physiotherapy Department of the Royal National Orthopaedic Hospital for their assistance with the chapters on Walking Aids and Crutch Walking. I also wish to express my gratitude to Professor R. G. Burwell who advised me on the original script, to Mr. J. Crawford Adams who read the final draft, and to Dr. R. R. Mason for his careful reading of the proofs.

JOHN D. M. STEWART.

Bognor Regis, 1974.

To
D.M.S.

Contents

1. Traction

General Principles and Methods of Application

When a limb is painful as a result of inflammation of a joint or a fracture of one of the bones, the controlling muscles contract simultaneously. This is called muscle spasm. The antagonistic muscles in a limb are not all equally powerful, with the result that when muscle spasm is present, the action of the more powerful muscles can produce a deformity which may seriously impair the future function of the limb.

Inflammation of the hip joint commonly results in a flexion, adduction and lateral rotation deformity, the presence of which causes apparent shortening of the affected lower limb.

When the shaft of the femur is fractured at the junction of the upper and middle thirds, the proximal fragment is flexed and abducted by the pull of the ilio-psoas and hip abductor muscles respectively, and the distal fragment is adducted by the adductor muscles of the thigh. In addition, if apposition of the fragments is lost, marked shortening of the femur occurs.

Traction, by overcoming muscle spasm, relieves pain and thus allows a limb to be rested in the best functional position. In addition, traction reduces the movement of an injured part of the body and thus aids in the healing of bone and soft tissues. When bony injury is present, the injured part is usually splinted.

METHODS OF APPLYING TRACTION

To apply traction, a satisfactory grip must be obtained on a part of the body. In the case of a limb, the traction force may be applied through the skin—*skin traction*—or via the bones—*skeletal traction*.

A traction force may be applied also to other parts of the body. Pelvic traction is described in Chapter 4, and spinal traction in Chapter 7.

Skin traction

The traction force is applied over a large area of skin. This spreads the load, and is more comfortable and efficient. In the treatment of fractures, the traction force must be applied only to the limb distal to the fracture site, otherwise the efficiency of the traction force is reduced.

The maximum traction weight which can be applied with skin traction is 15 lb (6·7 kg).

Two methods of applying skin traction are commonly used.

Adhesive strapping

This can only be stretched transversely. The necessary apparatus can be assembled individually, but prepared Elastoplast Skin Traction Kits (Smith and Nephew Ltd.)* for use in adults or children can be obtained.

Some patients are allergic to adhesive strapping. For these patients other preparations which do not utilize an adhesive containing zinc oxide can be used, for example Seton Skin Traction Kit (Seton Products Ltd.).* Two other preparations to which allergic reactions have not been reported are Orthotrac (Zimmer Orthopaedic Ltd.)* and Skin-Trac (Zimmer, U.S.A.).*

APPLICATION OF ADHESIVE STRAPPING

● Shave limb (shaving is not required with Orthotrac and Skin-Trac).
● Protect the malleoli from friction with a strip of felt, foam rubber or a few turns of bandage under the strapping.
● Starting at the ankle but leaving a loop projecting 4 to 6 inches (10 to 15 cm) beyond the sole of the foot, apply the widest possible strapping to both sides of the limb, parallel to a line between the lateral malleolus and the greater trochanter. On the lateral aspect the strapping must lie slightly behind, and on the medial aspect, slightly in front of this line to encourage medial rotation of the limb.
● Avoid wrinkles and creases. If necessary, nick the strapping to ensure that it lies flat.
● Avoid the malleoli, tibial crest and patella.
● Apply a crepe or elasticated bandage over the strapping, again starting at the ankle. A 6 inch (15 cm) bandage is used for adults, and a 4 inch (10 cm) bandage for children.
● Attach a spreader bar or cords to the distal end of the strapping.
● Attach the required traction weight.

Non-adhesive strapping

Ventfoam Skin Traction Bandage (The Scholl Manufacturing Co. Ltd.)* consists of lengths of soft, ventilated latex foam rubber laminated to a strong cloth backing. It is useful particularly on thin and atrophic skin, or when there is sensitivity to adhesive strapping. Its grip is less secure than that of adhesive strapping and therefore frequent reapplications may be necessary.

* See Appendix.

APPLICATION OF VENTFOAM SKIN TRACTION BANDAGE

Shaving of the limb is not required.

- Lie the Ventfoam Skin Traction Bandage (foam surface to the skin) on each side of the limb.
- Leave a loop projecting 4 to 6 inches (10 to 15 cm) beyond the sole of the foot.
- Apply a crepe bandage, beginning with 2 to 3 turns around the ankle under the Ventfoam Bandage before catching in each length. Continue bandaging up the limb over the Ventfoam Bandage.
- Place the metal spreader provided, in the loop formed.
- Attach a cord and the required traction weight to the metal spreader. The traction weight should not exceed 10 lb (4·5 kg).

Contraindications to skin traction

1. Abrasions of the skin.
2. Lacerations of the skin in the area to which the traction is to be applied.
3. Impairment of circulation—varicose ulcers, impending gangrene, stasis dermatitis.
4. Marked shortening of the bony fragments, when the traction weight required will be greater than can be applied through the skin.

Complications of skin traction

1. Allergic reactions to the adhesive.
2. Excoriation of the skin from slipping of the adhesive strapping.
3. Pressure sores around the malleoli and over the tendo calcaneus.
4. Common peroneal nerve palsy. This may result from two causes. Rotation of the limb is difficult to control with skin traction. There is a tendency for the limb to rotate laterally and for the common peroneal nerve to be compressed by the slings on which the limb rests. Adhesive strapping tends to slide slowly down the limb, carrying the encircling bandage with it. The circumference of the limb around the knee is greater than that around the head of the fibula. The downward slide of the adhesive strapping and bandage is halted at the head of the fibula. This can cause pressure on the common peroneal nerve.

Skeletal traction

For skeletal traction, a metal pin or wire is driven through the bone. By this means the traction force is applied directly to the skeleton. (For spinal traction, see Chapter 7.)

Skeletal traction is seldom necessary in the management of upper limb fractures. It is used frequently in the management of lower limb fractures. It may be employed as a means of reducing or of maintaining the reduction of a fracture. It should be reserved for those cases in which skin traction is contraindicated. A serious complication of skeletal traction is bony infection.

Steinmann pin

Steinmann pins (Steinmann, 1916) are rigid stainless steel pins of varying lengths, 4 to 6 millimetres in diameter. After insertion, a special stirrup (Böhler, 1929), illustrated in Figure 1.1, is attached to the pin. The Böhler stirrup allows the direction of the traction to be varied without turning the pin in the bone.

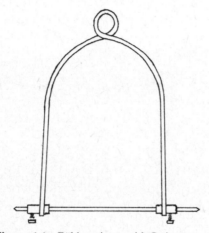

Figure 1.1   Böhler stirrup with Steinmann pin.

Denham pin

The Denham pin (Denham, 1972) illustrated in Figure 1.2, is identical to a Steinmann pin except for a short threaded length situated towards the end held in the introducer. This threaded portion engages the bony cortex and reduces the risk of the pin sliding. This type of pin is particularly suitable for use in cancellous bone, such as the calcaneus, or in osteoporotic bone.

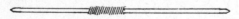

Figure 1.2   Denham pin.

Kirschner wire

A Kirschner wire (Kirschner, 1909) is of small diameter, and is insufficiently rigid until pulled taut in a special stirrup (Fig. 1.3) (Kirschner, 1927). Rotation of the stirrup is imparted to the wire. The wire easily cuts out of bone if a heavy traction weight is applied. Although Kirschner wires can be used in the lower limb, they are more often used in the upper limb.

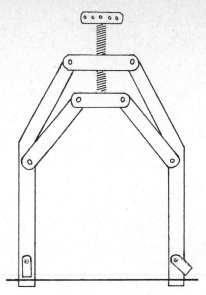

Figure 1.3   Kirschner wire strainer.

Common sites for application of skeletal traction

LOWER END OF FEMUR

Prolonged traction through the lower end of the femur predisposes to knee stiffness from fibrosis in the extensor mechanism of the knee. For this reason, a Steinmann pin through the lower end of the femur must be removed after two to three weeks and be replaced by one through the upper end of the tibia.

The point of insertion for skeletal traction through the lower end of the femur can be determined in two ways.

1. Draw a line from before backwards at the level of the upper pole of the patella. Draw a second line from below upwards anterior to the head of the fibula. Where these two lines intersect is the point of insertion of a Steinmann pin (Fig. 1.4).

2. Just proximal to the upper limit of the lateral femoral condyle. In the average adult this point is $1\frac{1}{4}$ inches (3·0 cm) proximal to the articulation between the lateral femoral condyle and the lateral tibial plateau.

Care must be taken to avoid entering the knee joint. The lateral fold of the capsule of the knee joint reaches $\frac{1}{2}$ to $\frac{3}{4}$ inch (1·25 to 2·0 cm) above the level of the joint (Fig. 1.4).

UPPER END OF TIBIA

The point of insertion is $\frac{3}{4}$ inch (2·0 cm) behind the crest, just below the level of the tubercle of the tibia (Fig. 1.4).

LOWER END OF TIBIA

The point of insertion is 2 inches (5·0 cm) above the level of the ankle joint, mid-way between the anterior and posterior borders of the tibia (Fig. 1.5).

CALCANEUS

The point of insertion is ¾ inch (2·0 cm) below and behind the lateral malleolus. (As the lateral malleolus lies ½ inch (1·25 cm) more posterior and distal than the medial malleolus, the above point corresponds with that 1¼ inches (3·0 cm) below and behind the medial malleolus). Care must be taken to avoid entering the subtalar joint (Fig. 1.5).

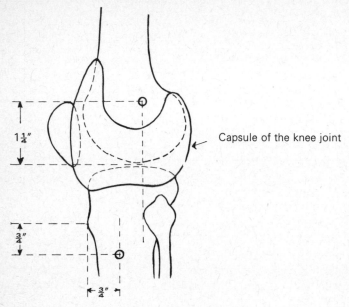

Figure 1.4   Position for Steinmann pin in lower end of femur and upper end of tibia.

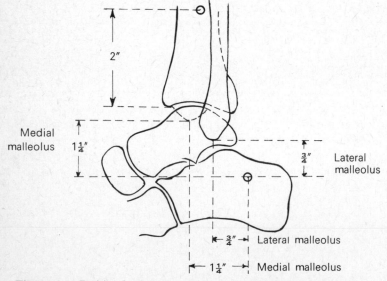

Figure 1.5   Position for Steinmann pin in lower end of tibia and calcaneus.

The insertion of a Steinmann pin through the calcaneus may result in stiffness of the subtalar joint, or more seriously, in infection in the bone. However, with a pin in this site, the traction force is applied in the line of the calf muscles, counteracts their pull, and thereby reduces the deforming action of these muscles on the fracture. When possible the lower tibial site for insertion of a Steinmann pin should be used.

APPLICATION OF SKELETAL TRACTION, USING A STEINMANN PIN

- Use general or local anaesthesia. If local anaesthesia is used, the skin and the periosteum must be infiltrated.
- Shave the skin.
- Use full aseptic precautions—mask, cap, gown, gloves and drapes.
- Paint the skin with iodine.
- Drape skin towels under and around the limb.
- Mount the Steinmann pin on the introducer.
- Ask an assistant to hold the ankle at a right angle, with the toes pointing straight upwards.
- Identify the site of insertion (see above).
- Hold the pin horizontally and at right angles to the long axis of the limb.
- Drive the pin from lateral to medial, through the skin and the bone with a gentle twisting motion of the forearm, while keeping the flexed elbow against the side of your body.
- Apply on each side a small cotton wool pad, soaked in Benzomastic, around the pin to seal the wounds. Always use two separate pads. One strip of gauze wound back and forth across the shin and around the Steinmann pin may cause a pressure sore. Benzomastic is the best sealing compound as it will stick to skin and metal.
- Fit the Böhler stirrup.
- Apply guards over the ends of the pin.

By not incising the skin with a scalpel prior to inserting the Steinmann pin, a much tighter fit around the pin is obtained, thus reducing the chances of infection and puckering of the skin on one side of the pin. If the skin does pucker, it should be incised and one or two sutures inserted if necessary.

A Steinmann pin may also be gently hammered in. It is inadvisable to use this method when inserting a pin into the lower end of the femur or tibia, as splintering of the cortex may occur.

COUNTER-TRACTION

One of the reasons for applying a traction force to a part of the body is to counteract the deforming effects of muscle spasm. The muscles in spasm tend to draw the distal part of the body in a proximal direction. A traction force applied to the affected part of the body will overcome muscle spasm only if another force acting in the opposite direction—*counter-traction*—is applied at the same time as the traction force. If counter-traction is not applied, the whole body will be pulled in the direction of the traction force, and muscle spasm will not be overcome.

Fixed traction

One method of obtaining counter-traction is by applying a force against a fixed point on the body, proximal to the attachments of the muscles in spasm. A similar situation exists when an attempt is made to extract a cork from a bottle. The neck of the bottle is gripped in one hand and the corkscrew in the other. When a traction force is *initially* applied to the corkscrew, another force, acting in the opposite direction (counter-traction), is applied at the same time to the bottle, the counter-traction force passing along the arm to the neck of the bottle. This mechanical arrangement is called *fixed traction*.

To apply a force against a fixed point on the body, an appliance, for example a Thomas's splint (see Chapter 2) is used. The ring of the splint snugly encircles the root of the limb. The traction cords are tied to the distal end of the splint, and the counter-traction force passes along the side bars of the splint to the ring and hence to the body proximal to the attachment of the muscles in spasm (Fig. 3.1).

Fixed traction is discussed in Chapter 3.

Sliding traction

Gravity may be utilized to provide counter-traction by tilting the bed so that the patient tends to slide in the opposite direction to that of the traction force. This is called *sliding traction* and is discussed in Chapter 4. A splint is often used when sliding traction is employed, but the function of the splint in this instance is merely to cradle the limb.

REFERENCES

BÖHLER, L. (1929) *The Treatment of Fractures.* English Translation by Steinberg, M. E. p. 38 and p. 39, Fig. 56. Vienna: W. Maudrich.
DENHAM, R. A. (1972) Personal communication.
KIRSCHNER, M. VON (1909): Ueber Nagelextension. *Beiträge zur Klinischen Chirurgie,* **64**, 266.
KIRSCHNER, M. VON (1927) Verbesserungen Der Drahtextension. *Archiv Für Klinische Chirurgie,* **148**, 651.
STEINMANN, F. VON (1916) Die Nagelextension. *Ergebnisse Der Chirurgie und Orthopädie,* **9**, 520.

2. The Thomas's and Fisk splints

THOMAS'S SPLINT

The splint which today is called the Thomas's splint was described originally by Hugh Owen Thomas (Thomas, 1876) as a knee appliance which he used in the ambulant management of chronic or subacute inflammation of the knee joint. The present splint consists of a padded oval metal ring covered with soft leather, to which are attached inner and outer side bars. These side bars which exactly bisect the oval ring, are of unequal length so that the padded ring is set at an angle of 120 degrees to the inner side bar. At the distal end the two side bars are joined together in the form of a 'W'. The outer side bar is often angled out 2 inches (5.0 cm) below the padded ring, to clear a prominent greater trochanter (Fig. 3.1).

The padded ring is made in different sizes and the side bars in varying lengths.

CHOOSING A THOMAS'S SPLINT
1. Measure the oblique circumference of the thigh immediately below the gluteal fold and ischial tuberosity. The line of measurement is oblique and must correspond with the inclination of the ring of the splint (Fig. 2.1). This measurement equals the *internal* circumference of the padded ring. If the above measurement cannot be taken without causing the patient pain, measure the oblique circumference of the normal thigh. Add 2 inches (5·0 cm) to this measurement if there is much swelling of the injured thigh. Accuracy is required if fixed traction is intended. With sliding traction, accuracy is not so important because the function of the splint is merely to support the limb.
2. Measure the distance from the crotch to the heel *and add 6 to 9 inches (15 to 23 cm)*. This distance equals the length of the inner side bar (Fig. 2.1).

PREPARING A THOMAS'S SPLINT
1. Fashion slings, between the side bars, on which the limb can rest.
- Cut an adequate length of 6 inch (15·0 cm) wide domette bandage or calico. It is better to cut off excess length later, than to have to change a sling which is too short, after the limb has been placed in the splint.
- Pass the length of domette bandage or calico around the inner side bar. Then pass *both ends above* the outer side bar (Fig. 2.2).

9

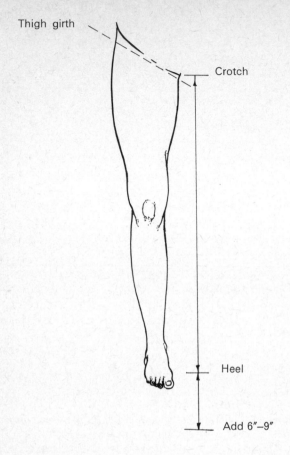

Figure 2.1   How to measure for a Thomas's splint.

● Fasten the two ends to the sling so formed with two large safety pins or toothed clips.

In this way the tension of the sling can be adjusted easily after the splint has been fitted to the limb (Fig. 2.2), to ensure uniform support

Figure 2.2   Detail of fixing of sling to inner and outer side bars of a Thomas's splint.

of the limb, and to avoid excess pressure in the region of the neck of the fibula and the tendo calcaneus.

The *proximal sling* leaves a triangular area of thigh unsupported because of the obliquity of the ring of the splint with the side bars. This triangular area can be supported by passing the length of domette bandage around the ring of the splint as well as the side bars (Fig. 2.3), (Strange, 1965).

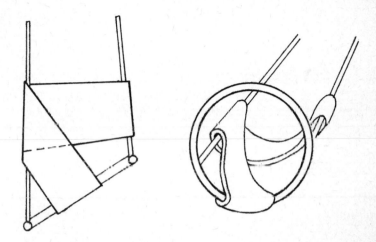

Figure 2.3 Method of arranging the proximal sling to obliterate the triangular gap which results from the obliquity of the ring of a Thomas's splint.

The *distal sling* must end 2½ inches (6·0 cm) above the heel to avoid pressure sores developing over the tendo calcaneus (Fig. 2.4).

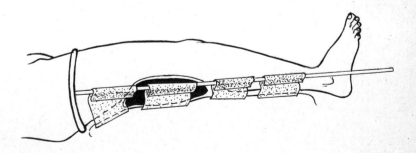

Figure 2.4 Arrangement of pad, slings and gamgee lining for a Thomas's splint.

The slings tend to slip distally on the side bars of the Thomas's splint. This can be prevented by pinning each sling to the one above or by binding the side bars with zinc oxide strapping before applying the slings.

A safe and comfortable substitute for domette slings is an elastic tube bandage (Tubigrip—Seton Products Ltd.*). A Tubigrip bandage is slipped over the splint, the ends are folded back, and the position held with safety pins. When an exceptionally heavy limb has to be supported, the thickness of the Tubigrip can be doubled (Board, 1967).

2. Line the slings with Gamgee tissue.

3. Fashion one large pad from Gamgee tissue or cotton wool. This pad should measure roughly 6 by 9 inches (15 by 23 cm) and be about 2 inches (5·0 cm) thick when compressed. Place this pad transversely under the lower part of the thigh to maintain the normal anterior bowing of the femoral shaft (Fig. 2.4).

4. If the leg is to be supported in a knee-flexion piece, the hinge must coincide with the axis of movement of the knee joint. The movement of flexion and extension at a normal knee joint is not one of simple hinge movement, but is complex, following a polycentric pathway (the instant centres determined for each increment of flexion moving posteriorly in a spiral pattern (Gunston, 1971), as shown in Fig. 2.5).

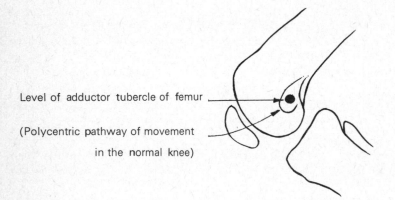

Level of adductor tubercle of femur

(Polycentric pathway of movement

in the normal knee)

Figure 2.5   Hinge of knee-flexion piece is sited level with the adductor tubercle of the femur.

However, from the point of view of the siting of the hinge of a knee-flexion piece, the axis of movement is taken to lie level with the adductor tubercle of the femur (Fig. 2.5).

5. After the splint has been fitted, bandage the limb into the splint.

* See Appendix.

FISK SPLINT

The splint described by Fisk (1944) consists of a modified Thomas's splint to which a knee-flexion piece is attached. The Thomas's splint is modified by removing the side bars beyond the level of the knee joint, and turning the cut ends of the side bars horizontally outwards to form small rings. A knee-flexion piece is fixed firmly to the side bars just proximal to these rings, level with the axis of movement of the knee joint.

The splint is now purpose-designed* (Fig. 2.6). The padded groin ring, the front half of which is replaced by a padded strap

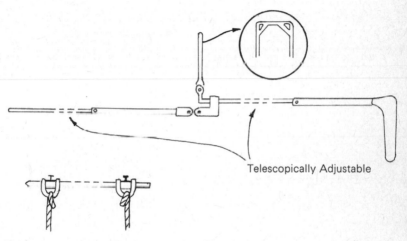

Figure 2.6 Fisk splint, side-view. Insert shows method used to attach traction cords to a Steinmann pin with locking collars and U-stirrups.

and buckle, is attached by swivel joints to the side bars, so that the same splint can be used for either limb. The distal ends of the side bars are connected just beyond the knee by a squared-off frame which has two small eyelets at each upper corner. The knee-flexion piece is fixed to the side bars, just proximal to the squared-off frame, through off-set double-cog hinges. These hinges must lie at the level of the axis of movement of the knee joint when the splint is applied to the limb. The side bars of the thigh and knee-flexion parts of the splint are adjustable telescopically, thus enabling all lengths of lower limb to be accommodated.

Application of sliding traction with the Fisk splint is described in Chapter 4, and suspension of the splint in Chapter 5.

---

* See Appendix.

REFERENCES

BOARD, C. P. (1967) Sling for Thomas's splint. *Lancet*, **ii**, 757.

FISK, G. R. (1944) The fractured femoral shaft: new approach to the problem. *Lancet*, **i**, 659.

GUNSTON, F. H. (1971) Polycentric knee arthroplasty. *Journal of Bone and Joint Surgery*, **53-B**, 272.

STRANGE, F. G. St. C. (1965) *The Hip*, p. 99, Fig. iv.6 and p. 269, Fig. x.7. London: Heinemann.

THOMAS, H. O. (1876) *Diseases of the Hip, Knee and Ankle Joints, with Their Deformities, Treated by a New and Efficient Method*, 2nd ed., p. 98 and Plate 13, Fig. 4. Liverpool: T. Dobb & Co.

3. Fixed traction

If traction is applied to a limb, counter-traction acting in the opposite direction must be applied also, to prevent the body from being pulled in the direction of the traction force. When counter-traction acts through an appliance which obtains a purchase on a part of the body, the arrangement is called fixed traction.

FIXED TRACTION IN A THOMAS'S SPLINT

Fixed traction in a Thomas's splint can 'maintain', but *not* 'obtain' the reduction of a fracture. It is therefore indicated when the femoral fracture can be reduced by manipulation. A reduced transverse fracture is most suitable, but the reduction of an oblique or spiral fracture can be maintained also.

When the cords attached to the adhesive strapping or a tibial Steinmann pin are pulled tight, the counter-thrust passes up the side bars of the splint to the padded ring around the root of the limb (Fig. 3.1). The ring, which must be a snug fit, may cause pressure sores unless daily attention is paid to the skin (see Chapter 6). The pressure of the padded ring around the root of the limb can be reduced partly by pulling on the end of the splint. A traction weight of 5 lb (2·3 kg) attached to the Thomas's splint usually is sufficient for this purpose.

The significant feature of fixed traction is that the traction force balances the pull of the muscles and, as the muscular pull and haematoma decrease, the traction force decreases. Distraction at the fracture site and the accompanying danger of delayed union or non-union of the fracture is less likely to occur. It is not necessary in this system repeatedly to tighten the traction cords with a windlass, except to compensate for any stretching of the cords or sliding downwards of the adhesive strapping if skin traction is employed.

As counter-traction is not dependant upon gravity the apparatus is self-contained, and the patient may be lifted and moved without risk of displacement of the fracture. This method is valuable in the treatment of civilian casualties. During the Second World War a modification of this method was employed. The whole limb and the Thomas's splint was encased in plaster-of-Paris; this assembly was known as the Tobruk splint (Bristow, 1943).

15

For comfort and ease of movement of the patient, the Thomas's splint can be suspended (see Chapter 5).

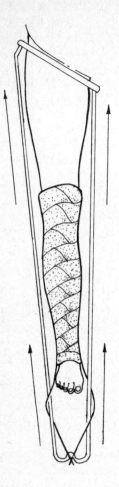

Figure 3.1

Fixed traction in a Thomas's splint. The grip on the leg is obtained by adhesive strapping.

Note :—the ring of the Thomas's splint is well up in the groin and fits snugly around the root of the limb.

—the malleoli are well padded to avoid pressure.

—the outer traction cord passes above and the inner cord passes below its respective side bar, to hold the limb in medial rotation.

—the traction cords are tied over the end of the Thomas's splint.

—a windlass is omitted. This avoids the temptation to repeatedly tighten the traction cords and thereby either distract the fracture or pull the adhesive strapping off the limb.

—the counter thrust (traction) passes up the side bars, as indicated by the arrows, to the root of the limb.

REDUCTION OF A FEMORAL SHAFT FRACTURE

For children skin traction is adequate, but for adults skeletal traction with an upper tibial Steinmann pin (Denham pin for the elderly) is used more frequently.

● Insert an upper tibial Steinmann pin under general anaesthesia and attach a Böhler stirrup.

● Thread the prepared Thomas's splint over the limb.

● Palpate the dorsalis pedis and posterior tibial pulses.

● Study the radiographs. Determine the type of fracture, in which direction the fragments are displaced and in which direction they need to be moved to obtain apposition of the bone ends. The next step depends upon the type of fracture.

Transverse fracture. An assistant standing at the foot of the splint holds the Böhler stirrup, exerts a traction force in the long axis of the limb, and simultaneoulsy forces the ring of the splint against the ischial tuberosity.

- Stand at the side of the limb and grip the limb above and below the fracture site. Move the proximal and distal fragments in the directions determined from the study of the pre-reduction radiographs, to reduce the fracture. For example, in a fracture at the junction of the middle and lower thirds of the shaft of the femur, the distal fragment usually is displaced posteriorly. Therefore place one hand under the distal fragment and the other on top of the proximal fragment, and push anteriorly with the hand under the distal fragment. The general rule is that the distal fragment is reduced to the proximal fragment and not vice versa, as the manipulator has control only of the distal fragment, the proximal fragment being under control of the muscles attached to it.
- Check that apposition of the fragments has been obtained by temporarily reducing the traction force. The absence of telescoping of the limb indicates that apposition has been achieved.
- When apposition has been obtained, carefully lower the limb, while maintaining traction, onto the prepared Thomas's splint, with the large pad under the lower part of the thigh.
- Maintain traction.
- Arrange the tension in the other slings to allow 15 to 20 degrees of knee flexion.
- Attach traction cords to each end of the Steinmann pin and tie them to the lower end of the Thomas's splint.
- Release the pull on the Böhler stirrup.
- Take antero-posterior and lateral radiographs to check the reduction of the fracture. If the reduction is not satisfactory, re-manipulate.
- Palpate the dorsalis pedis and posterior tibial pulses. If the pulses are absent, reduce the traction force. If the pulses do not return, *very gently* re-manipulate the fracture. *If the peripheral pulses are still absent, notify more senior colleagues immediately.*
- If the peripheral pulses are present and the reduction is satisfactory, remove the Böhler stirrup.
- Suspend the Thomas's splint (see Chapter 5).

Oblique, spiral or comminuted fractures. A formal manipulation of these fractures is not required. The traction force is applied in the long axis of the limb as described above, until the fractured femur is restored to its correct length. Traction is maintained until the traction cords are tied to the foot of the Thomas's splint.

The instructions about the large pad, radiographs, peripheral pulses and suspension of the Thomas's splint also apply.

Traction unit

For many years, Charnley (1970), has employed what he terms a traction unit (Fig. 3.2), in conjunction with fixed traction in a Thomas's splint, for the management of fractures of the femoral shaft. Basically a traction unit consists of an upper tibial Steinmann pin incorporated in a light below-knee plaster cast.

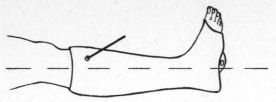

Figure 3.2   Traction unit. The broken line shows the position of the side bars of the Thomas's splint in relation to the cross-bar fixed to the sole of the plaster cast.

APPLICATION OF A TRACTION UNIT WITH FIXED TRACTION
- Choose the correct size of Thomas's splint.
- Fashion one sling and a large pad to support the thigh.
- Under general anaesthesia, thread the prepared Thomas's splint over the limb, insert an upper tibial Steinmann pin and attach a Böhler stirrup.
- While the leg is supported by an assistant holding the stirrup and keeping the foot at a right angle, apply a padded below-knee plaster cast incorporating the Steinmann pin. The cast must be well padded around the heel to prevent pressure sores from developing.
- Incorporate a 6 inch (15·0 cm) long wooden bar transversely in the sole of the plaster cast about mid-way between the heel and the toes. This bar controls rotation of the limb.
- When the plaster cast has hardened, reduce the fracture and lower the limb onto the prepared splint.
- Check that the thigh sling and the large pad correctly support the thigh, maintaining the normal anterior bowing of the femoral shaft.
- Allow the transverse bar to rest on the side bars of the Thomas's splint. If the thigh sling is correctly tensioned, and the transverse bar is positioned correctly, the knee should be in 15 to 20 degrees of flexion, and the limb in neutral rotation.
- Attach a cord to each end of the Steinmann pin, loop them once around the side bars of the splint and tie them over the end of the splint.
- Check that the pressure of the thigh sling against the thigh is not excessive. If it is, reduce the pressure by placing a sling under the upper end of the traction unit. The tighter the calf sling is pulled, the more the pressure on the thigh is relieved.
- Suspend the Thomas's splint (Charnley uses Method 2, Chapter 5).
- Attach a 5 lb (2·3 kg) weight to the end of the Thomas's splint to reduce partly the pressure of the padded ring of the splint around the root of the limb.

Advantages of the traction unit
1. Compression of the tissues of the upper calf, in particular the common peroneal nerve, does not occur. When fixed traction without a traction unit is employed, the upper calf may be com-

pressed between the Steinmann pin and the upper edge of the sling supporting the calf. Even when a sling is used to support the traction unit, compression of the calf does not occur because it is protected by the plaster cast.

2. Equinus deformity at the ankle cannot occur because the foot is supported by the plaster cast.
3. The tendo calcaneus is protected from pressure by the padded cast.
4. Rotation of the foot and the distal fragment is controlled.
5. A fracture of the ipsilateral tibia can be treated conservatively at the same time as the femoral fracture.

ROGER ANDERSON WELL-LEG TRACTION

Well-leg traction (Anderson, 1932) was originally used in the management of fractures of the pelvis, femur and tibia, skeletal traction being applied to the injured leg, while the 'well' leg was employed for counter-traction. It is rarely used for these purposes today. This method however is valuable in correcting either an abduction or adduction deformity at the hip, for instance before an extra-articular arthrodesis is carried out.

The principle is as follows:

With an abduction deformity at the hip, the affected limb appears to be longer. When traction is applied to the 'well' limb and the affected limb is simultaneously pushed up (counter-traction), the abduction deformity is reduced. Reversing the arrangement will reduce an adduction deformity (Fig. 3.3).

ADDUCTION
DEFORMITY

ABDUCTION
DEFORMITY

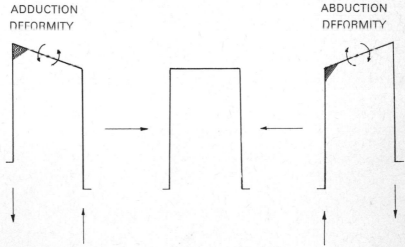

Figure 3.3 Diagramatic illustration of the principle of Roger Anderson well-leg traction.

APPLICATION OF ROGER ANDERSON WELL-LEG TRACTION

The simultaneous pulling down of one leg and the pushing up of the other is achieved by using the apparatus illustrated in Figure 3.4.

Line of iliac spines ——

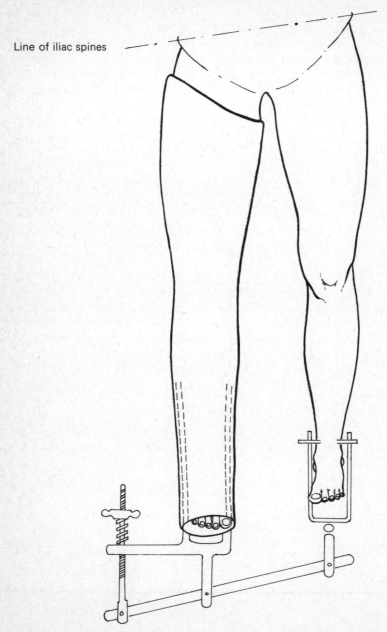

Figure 3.4 Roger Anderson well-leg traction (modified). The padded below-knee plaster cast is not illustrated.

- Apply an above-knee plaster cast to the limb which is to be pushed upwards. This plaster cast must extend to the top of the thigh; it must be well padded and moulded over the medial aspect of the upper thigh, to prevent the cast pressing on the tissues and obstructing the circulation; and it must be well padded around the ankle and heel as these will be the sites of continuous pressure from the direction of the heel.
- Incorporate the larger stirrup in this plaster.
- Insert a Steinmann pin through the lower end of the tibia of the limb which is to be pulled down, and incorporate the Steinmann pin in a light padded below-knee plaster cast.
- Pass the ends of the Steinmann pin through the lowest possible holes in the side arms of the smaller stirrup.

By altering the position of the screw (on the left in Figure 3.4), the relative positions of the two stirrups can be altered.

The arrangement illustrated in Figure 3.4 can be used to correct an abduction deformity at the right hip, or an adduction deformity at the left hip.

REFERENCES

ANDERSON, R. (1932) A new method of treating fractures, utilizing the well leg for counter traction. *Surgery, Gynaecology and Obstetrics*, 54, 207.

BRISTOW, W. R. (1943) Some surgical lessons of the war. *Journal of Bone and Joint Surgery*, 25, 524.

CHARNLEY, J. (1970) *The Closed Treatment of Common Fractures*, 3rd ed., p. 179. Edinburgh and London: Churchill Livingstone.

4. Sliding traction

In 1839, John Haddy James of Exeter described a method, which he had employed for several years, of treating fractures of the lower limb with 'continuous yet tolerable traction . . . by weight and pulley' (Jones, 1953). The patient's trunk was fixed to the head of the bed by a rib bandage. The leg was bandaged into a padded hollow splint fitted with a foot piece. A castor on the hollow splint rested upon a wooden plank. A cord from the footpiece passed over a pulley at the foot of the bed to a weight. The head of the bed was raised. James did not utilize the weight of the body, acting under the influence of gravity, to provide counter-traction. In his system, counter-traction was represented by the tension in the rib bandage.

When the weight of all or part of the body, acting under the influence of gravity, is utilized to provide counter-traction, the arrangement is called sliding traction. The traction force is applied by a weight, attached to adhesive strapping or a steel pin by a cord acting over a pulley (Fig. 4.1). The traction force continues to act as long as the weight remains clear of the floor. Counter-traction is obtained by raising one end of the bed by means of wooden blocks or a bed elevator, so that the body tends to slide in the opposite direction to that of the traction force.

When sliding traction is used to reduce a fracture, the initial traction weight required to obtain the reduction is greater than the traction weight required to maintain the reduction. *Great care must be taken to ensure that distraction of the fracture does not occur.* For

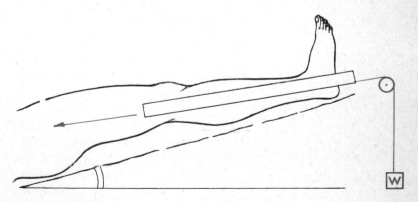

Figure 4.1   The principle of sliding traction.

this reason the length of the fractured bone must be measured daily with a tape measure and compared with the normal side, until the correct length has been obtained. When this has been achieved, the traction weight must be reduced to that sufficient to maintain the reduction. Daily radiographic examination may be employed, *but do not ignore the use of a tape measure.*

The traction weight needed to reduce or to maintain the reduction of a particular fracture depends upon the site of the fracture, the age and weight of the patient, the power of his muscles, the amount of muscle damage present and the degree of friction present in the system. The exact weight required is determined by trial, and observing the behaviour of the fracture. For a fracture of the femoral shaft an initial weight of 10 to 20 lb (4·5 to 9·0 kg) is usually sufficient for an average adult, and 2 to 10 lb (1·0 to 4·5 kg) for an average child. The heavier the traction weight used, the higher the end of the bed must be raised to provide adequate counter-traction.

BUCK'S TRACTION OR EXTENSION

Buck's traction, popularised during the American Civil War (Buck, 1861), is used in the temporary management of fractures of the femoral neck and in the management of fractures of the femoral shaft in older and larger children.

APPLICATION OF BUCK'S TRACTION
- Apply adhesive strapping to above the knee or, in elderly patients, with atrophic skin, Ventfoam Skin Traction Bandage.
- Support the leg on a soft pillow to keep the heel clear of the bed.
- Pass the cord from the spreader over a pulley attached to the end of the bed.
- Attach 5 to 7 lb (2·3 to 3·2 kg) to the cord.
- Elevate the foot of the bed.
     Lateral rotation of the limb is not controlled by this method of traction.

SLIDING TRACTION WITH A THOMAS'S SPLINT AND A KNEE-FLEXION PIECE

Sliding traction in a Thomas's splint with a knee-flexion piece (Fig. 4.2) is often employed to obtain the reduction of an oblique or spiral fracture of the shaft of the femur, and then to retain that reduction until union occurs. The use of a knee-flexion piece allows easier mobilisation of the knee. In addition knee flexion controls rotation, prevents stretching of the posterior capsule and posterior

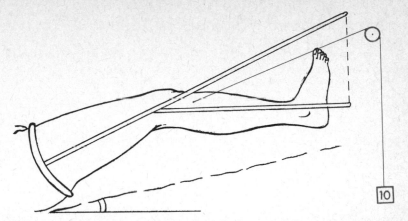

Figure 4.2 Sliding traction—skeletal. The lower limb rests in a Thomas's splint and knee-flexion piece. A Steinmann pin is inserted through the upper end of the tibia. A traction cord passes from the pin over a pulley to the traction weight. The foot of the bed is raised to provide counter-traction.

cruciate ligament of the knee, which might cause hyperextension instability, and allows variation in the direction of pull when a tibial Steinmann pin is used.

APPLICATION OF SLIDING TRACTION WITH A THOMAS'S SPLINT AND KNEE-FLEXION PIECE

- Choose the correct size of Thomas's splint (see Chapter 2).
- Fashion slings on the knee-flexion piece and the proximal part of the Thomas's splint, and line the slings with Gamgee tissue.
- Insert an upper tibial Steinmann pin.
- Pass the prepared Thomas's splint over the limb, and rest the limb on the padded slings. Remember the large pad under the lower part of the thigh.
- Check that the hinge of the knee-flexion piece lies at the level of the adductor tubercle of the femur.
- Suspend the distal end of the knee-flexion piece by two cords, one on each side, from the distal end of the Thomas's splint. The length of cord is such that the knee is flexed 20 to 30 degrees. (The extended position is regarded as zero degrees and flexion is measured from this starting position—American Academy of Orthopaedic Surgeons, 1965). With a supracondylar fracture of the femur, the distal fragment is usually tilted anteriorly upon the shaft. To correct anterior tilting, knee flexion is increased, the amount of knee flexion required being determined radiographically. The end of the knee-flexion piece may be suspended independently by a cord attached to a weight (see Chapter 5). This arrangement allows greater freedom of knee movement.
- Suspend the Thomas's splint (see Chapter 5).
- Adjust the position of the thigh pad and the tension in the sling supporting the pad to obtain the normal anterior bowing of the femoral shaft.

- Bandage the thigh into the Thomas's splint.
- Attach a Böhler stirrup and cord to the Steinmann pin.
- Pass the cord over a pulley at the foot of the bed so that the cord is in line with the shaft of the femur.
- Attach a weight to the cord.
- Elevate the foot of the bed.

SLIDING TRACTION WITH A 'FIXED' THOMAS'S SPLINT

When sliding traction with a Thomas's splint is employed in the treatment of a fracture of the shaft of the femur, there is a tendency for the splint to slip down the limb. This can be avoided by the careful arrangement of the suspension cords (see Chapter 5) or by fixing the traction cords from the patient to the splint, and then pulling on the splint. By this means the traction force passes via the splint to the lower limb (Strange, 1972). A knee-flexion piece is not used.

APPLICATION OF SLIDING TRACTION WITH A 'FIXED' THOMAS'S SPLINT (Strange, 1972)
See Figure 4.3.
- Choose the correct size of Thomas's splint (see Chapter 2).
- Pass the Thomas's splint over the limb while maintaining gentle manual traction.
- Under local or general anaesthesia, insert a Kirschner wire or Steinmann pin through the upper end of the tibia. When a Kirschner wire is used, it must be tensioned with the special Kirschner wire strainer (Fig. 1.3) using right-angled washers. The Kirschner wire strainer must be kept vertical. If it is allowed to lie on the crest of the tibia even for only a short time, a pressure sore will develop.
- Insert 'S' hooks with cords attached into the holes in the right-angled washers.
- Twist the cords twice around the side bars of the Thomas's splint.

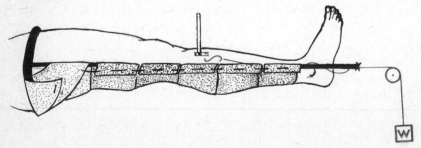

Figure 4.3 Sliding traction with a 'fixed' Thomas's splint. Note that the Kirschner wire strainer must be kept vertical (Strange, 1972).

- Push the Thomas's splint into the groin as far as possible and at the same time apply gentle steady traction to the cords. This achieves the optimal position.
- Tie the cords over the distal end of the Thomas's splint using a reef knot.
- Loop two pieces of tape around each side bar of the Thomas's splint, onc at the padded ring, and the other level with the foot.
- Fashion slings of domette (see Chapter 2) and adjust the tension in the slings to maintain the normal anterior bowing of the shaft of the femur and uniform support of the limb. A thigh pad may be used to maintain the anterior bowing of the shaft of the femur, but its use is not essential.
- Tie a traction cord to the end of the Thomas's splint using a clove hitch, then pass the cord over a pulley at the foot of the bed and attach it to a spring clip.
- Clip a weight to the traction cord. A weight of 18 lb (8·2 kg) is adequate for most adults.
- Suspend the Thomas's splint (see Chapter 5, Method 4) so that the heel is just off the bed, and the traction cord is in line with the splint.
- Elevate the foot of the bed.

SLIDING TRACTION IN A FISK SPLINT

The treatment of fractures of the femoral shaft and tibial condyles with sliding traction in a Fisk splint (Fig. 2.6) differs from other conservative methods (Fisk, 1944). With fixed traction in a Thomas's splint the knee is held in almost full extension, and little movement is possible. With sliding traction in a Thomas's splint with a knee-flexion piece, some active flexion and extension of the knee is possible, but little movement occurs at the hip, which is in flexion. When a Fisk splint is used, the patient, as soon as possible, begins assisted movement of the lower limb, which is moved as one unit as though the patient were walking. Passive movements are not encouraged (see Chapter 5).

Inhibition of muscular contraction is usually present for the first few days, but within two to three weeks powerful contractions are established. While the limb is exercised, variations in the line of the traction cord relative to the long axis of the femur, and angulation at the fracture site occur, but neither appear to adversely influence the result. Clinical union is present at four to six weeks and sound bony union occurs commonly by twelve weeks at which time a wide range of movement at the knee is present.

APPLICATION OF SLIDING TRACTION WITH A FISK SPLINT

- Adjust the splint to accommodate the limb (see Chapter 2).
- Fashion slings to support the thigh and calf.

- Insert an upper tibial Steinmann pin under general anaesthesia for fractures of the femur. Use skin traction for fractures of the tibial condyles.
- Attach a traction cord to each end of the Steinmann pin (Fig. 5.10) and tie these cords, which must be long enough to clear the foot, to a transverse wooden rod about 6 inches (15·0 cm) long.
- Pass the prepared splint over the limb.
- Manipulate the fracture (see Chapter 3).
- Adjust the position of the thigh pad to maintain the normal anterior bowing of the femoral shaft.
- Tie a single cord to the centre of the wooden rod, pass the cord over a pulley at the foot of the bed and attach a weight. After six weeks the initial traction weight is reduced to 6 to 8 lb (2·7 to 3·6 kg).
- Suspend the Fisk splint (see Chapter 5).
- Check that the traction cord is in line with the shaft of the femur (when a Steinmann pin is used) when the splint is suspended and the hip is flexed 45 degrees.
- Elevate the foot of the bed.

HAMILTON RUSSELL TRACTION

Hamilton Russell traction (Russell, 1924) is used in the management of fractures of the femoral shaft and after arthroplasty operations on the hip.

APPLICATION OF HAMILTON RUSSELL TRACTION
See Figure 4.4.
- Apply skin traction to the limb below the knee.
- Attach a pulley to the spreader.
- Place a soft broad sling under the knee.
- Support the limb, with the knee slightly flexed, on two soft pillows, one above and the other below the knee, with the heel clear of the bed.
- Attach a length of cord to the knee-sling.
- Pass the cord over pulley A which is placed well distal to, *not* proximal to the knee, round one of the pulleys B, round pulley C and then around the other pulley B before attaching it to a weight. The pulleys B must be at the same level as the foot of the patient when the leg is lying horizontally on a pillow (Fig. 4.4).
- Elevate the foot of the bed.
  Suggested weights :
  Adults—8 lb (3·6 kg).
  Infants and older children—½ to 4 lb (0·28 to 1·8 kg).

Theory of Hamilton Russell traction (Fig. 4.5)
The two pulley blocks B at the foot of the bed nominally double the pull on the limb. In practice the pull is modified by the friction present in the system. The resultant of the two forces acting along the cords provides a pull in the line of the shaft of the femur.

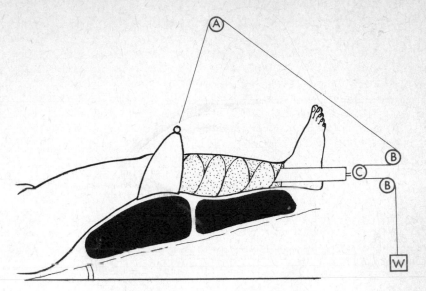

Figure 4.4   Hamilton Russell traction.

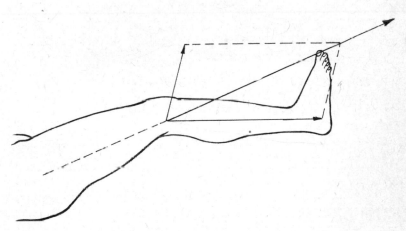

Figure 4.5   Theory of Hamilton Russell traction. The construction of a parallelogram of forces shows that the resultant force acts in the line of the femoral shaft.

TULLOCH BROWN TRACTION

Tulloch Brown, or U-loop tibial pin, traction and suspension (Nangle, 1951) with a Nissen foot plate and stirrup (Nissen, 1971), is used for the management of patients who have had a cup arthroplasty or pseudarthrosis operation on the hip, or who have sustained a fracture of the shaft of the femur. It is not used in children.

APPLICATION OF TULLOCH BROWN TRACTION

See Figure 4.6.

- Insert a Steinmann pin through the upper end of the tibia.
- Support the leg on slings suspended from the light duralumin U-loop which is slipped over the ends of the Steinmann pin.

Note : The proximal ends of the U-loop have two staggered lines of holes (Figs. 4.6 and 4.8). This arrangement gives a wide choice in the mode of attachment of the U-loop to the Steinmann pin. By varying the holes used, it is possible to ensure that the U-loop lies evenly on each side of the leg.

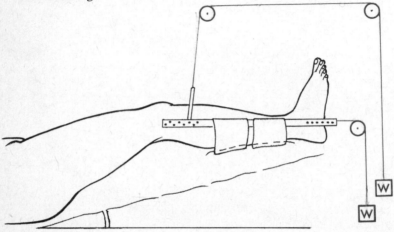

Figure 4.6   Tulloch Brown U-loop tibial pin traction. Alternatively the traction cords can be arranged as for Hamilton Russell traction (Fig. 4.4). A Nissen foot plate can be attached to the U-loop to maintain dorsiflexion at the ankle.

Care must be taken that the slings supporting the calf are not tight, otherwise compression of the tissues of the leg will occur between the proximal edge of the sling nearest the knee, and the Steinmann pin.

- Attach the Nisson stirrup (Fig. 4.7) to the Steinmann pin. This stirrup enables the leg to be suspended and rotation of the limb to be controlled.
- Mount the detachable Perspex foot plate on the U-loop to support the foot (Fig. 4.8). The foot plate prevents equinus of the ankle. In addition, as the attachment of the foot plate to the U-loop is not rigid, the leg muscles can be exercised.
- Use a simple pulley (Fig. 4.6) or Hamilton Russell system (Fig. 4.4) for suspension.
- Elevate the foot of the bed.

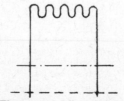

Figure 4.7   Nissen stirrup.

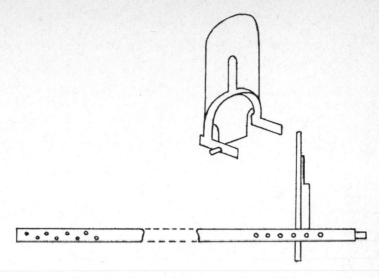

Figure 4.8   Detail of Nissen foot plate and U-loop.

BRYANT'S (OR GALLOWS) TRACTION (Fig. 4.9)

Bryant's traction (Bryant, 1880) is convenient and satisfactory for the treatment of fractures of the shaft of the femur in children up to the age of two years. Over this age, vascular complications, which are discussed later, may occur.

APPLICATION OF BRYANT'S TRACTION
- Apply adhesive strapping to *both* lower limbs (shaving is not necessary).
- (See below about the use of posterior gutter splints.)
- Tie the traction cords to an overhead beam.
- Tighten the traction cords sufficiently to raise the child's buttocks just clear of the mattress. Counter-traction is obtained by the weight of the pelvis and lower trunk.

Children tolerate this position very well, and good alignment of the fracture is obtained. When treating a fracture of the shaft of the femur in a young child, it is preferable to allow the fragments to overlap about ½ inch (1·25 cm), as subsequent overgrowth in length of the femur occurs due to hyperaemia of the limb consequent upon the fracture.

Fractures in children unite rapidly. It is therefore seldom necessary to maintain traction for more than four weeks.

Important : check the state of the circulation in the limbs frequently, because of the danger of vascular complications (see below).

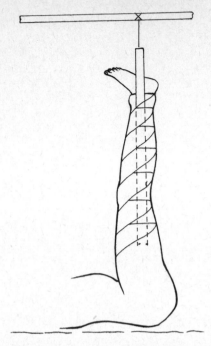

Figure 4.9   Bryant's (gallows) traction. Note: Child's buttocks are lifted just off the bed. Knees can be kept slightly flexed by applying posterior gutter splints (not illustrated).

Vascular complications of Bryant's traction

A careful check must be kept upon the state of the circulation in *both limbs*, especially during the first 24 to 72 hours after the application of the traction, because vascular complications may occur in either the injured or the normal limb.

HOW TO CHECK THE STATE OF THE CIRCULATION
- Observe the colour and temperature of *both feet*.
- Dorsiflex *both ankles* passively. *Dorsiflexion should be full and painless.* If dorsiflexion is limited or painful, muscle ischaemia may be present, therefore *lower the limbs and remove all bandaging and adhesive strapping immediately.*

A number of authors (Thompson and Mahoney, 1951; Miller *et al.*, 1952; Nicholson *et al.*, 1955; and Lidge, 1959) have reported vascular complications, varying from ischaemic fibrosis of the calf muscles to frank gangrene, following the use of Bryant's traction in children aged 3 to 8 years.

Nicholson *et al.* (1955) recorded the blood pressure at the ankles of children aged 1 to 8 years whose lower limbs were in the position as for Bryant's traction. They found a permanent reduction in the blood pressure at the ankles, which was in almost direct proportion to the hydrostatic pressure necessary to maintain a column of water at the height of the ankles above the heart. This reduction in the blood pressure was particularly proportional in children over the age of two years.

These authors also investigated the influence of hyperextension at the knees on the blood pressure at the ankles. They found, in children under the age of two years, that hyperextension at the knees with or without traction and irrespective of the position of the lower limbs, did not have any appreciable effect upon the blood pressure. In children over the age of 4 years however, the blood pressure at the ankles was reduced to zero when traction was applied with the knees hyperextended and when the lower limbs, without traction but with the knees hyperextended, were raised to the vertical.

Nicholson *et al.* (1955) concluded that in Bryant's traction the blood pressure at the ankles in children under the age of 2 years is insignificantly affected even with hyperextension at the knees; that between the ages of 2 and 4 years the circulation is precarious; and over the age of 4 years the circulation is definitely impaired.

Lidge (1959) stated that the use of Bryant's traction should be limited to children under 4 years old and to those weighing less than 35 to 40 lb (15·9 to 18·2 kg).

The use of Bryant's traction is reasonably safe in children under the age of 2 years. Between the ages of 2 to 4 years vascular complications are more likely to occur, but their occurrence is less likely if posterior gutter splints are applied to keep the knees in slight flexion. Over the age of 4 years the use of Bryant's traction is absolutely contraindicated.

In older children fractures of the shaft of the femur may be adequately treated in Buck's traction or in still older and larger children by fixed traction in a suspended Thomas's splint.

MODIFIED BRYANT'S TRACTION

Modified Bryant's traction is sometimes used in the initial management of congenital dislocation of the hip when diagnosed over the age of one year. Bryant's traction is set up as described above. After five days abduction of both hips is begun, abduction being increased by about 10 degrees on alternate days. By three weeks the hips should be fully abducted.

IMPORTANT
1. Check the state of the circulation as described above.
2. Occasionally, after an increase in the degree of abduction of the hips, the child will become restless and scream repeatedly with pain. The pain results from stretching of the capsule of the hip joint by impingement of the femoral head on the superior lip of the acetabulum. This occurs when abduction is commenced before the femoral head has been pulled down to lie opposite the acetabulum. Decreasing the degree of abduction will relieve the pain.

SLIDING TRACTION WITH A BÖHLER-BRAUN FRAME

Sliding traction with a Böhler-Braun frame (Böhler, 1929) can be used for the management of fractures of the tibia or femur. It is more commonly used on the continent of Europe. Although skin traction can be employed, skeletal traction is usually used.

The Böhler-Braun frame is illustrated in Fig. 4.10. Also indicated are the pulleys over which the cords pass when a femoral or tibial fracture is treated.

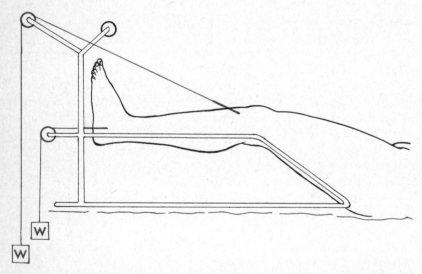

Figure 4.10   Böhler-Braun frame, showing the pulleys which are used when treating femoral or tibial fractures.

APPLICATION OF SLIDING TRACTION WITH A BÖHLER-BRAUN FRAME

● Suspend slings between the horizontal sides of the frame to support the thigh and leg. Cover the slings with Gamgee tissue.
● Insert a Steinmann pin through the upper end of the tibia for a femoral

fracture, or through the lower end of the tibia or the calcaneus for a tibial fracture.

● Attach a Böhler stirrup to the Steinmann pin.
● Place the limb on the slings.
● Attach a cord to the stirrup and pass the cord over the required pulley as shown in Figure 4.10.
● Attach a 7 to 10 lb (3·2 to 4·5 kg) weight to the cord.
● Elevate the foot of the bed.

This method of traction has certain disadvantages. The Böhler-Braun frame rests on the patient's bed, and cannot move with the patient. Nursing care is more difficult because the patient is not as mobile as he would be for example in a Thomas's splint. The patient's body and the proximal fragment of the fracture can move relative to the distal fragment which is cradled in the splint and is therefore relatively immobile. This may predispose to the occurrence of a deformity at the fracture site.

PELVIC TRACTION

In pelvic traction a special canvas harness is buckled around the patient's pelvis. Long cords or straps attach the harness to the foot of the bed. When the foot of the bed is raised, gravity causes the patient to slide towards the head of the bed. The amount by which the foot of the bed must be elevated depends upon the patient's weight: the heavier the patient, the more the foot of the bed must be raised.

This type of traction is used often in the conservative management of a prolapsed lumbar intervertebral disc. The function of the traction is to ensure that the patient lies quietly in bed, rather than to attempt to distract the vertebral bodies. The vertebral bodies can be distracted by traction, but the pull required is very much greater than that which can be exerted by this arrangement.

Buck's traction, applied to both lower limbs, with the cords attached either to the foot of the bed, or to traction weights, may be employed also in the conservative management of a prolapsed lumbar intervertebral disc. Pelvic traction is superior, however, because it leaves the patient's legs unencumbered and therefore able to move freely.

REFERENCES

AMERICAN ACADEMY OF ORTHOPAEDIC SURGEONS (1965) *Joint Motion: Method of Measuring and Recording* p. 66. Reprinted 1966 by The Orthopaedic Association. Edinburgh and London: Churchill Livingstone.

BÖHLER, L. (1929) *The Treatment of Fractures*. English Translation by Steinberg, M. E., p. 34 and p. 35, Fig. 48. Vienna: W. Maudrich.

REFERENCES *(continued)*

BRYANT, T. (1880) On the value of parallelism of the lower extremities in the treatment of hip disease and hip injuries, with the best means of obtaining it. *Lancet*, **i**, 159.

BUCK, G. (1861) An improved method of treating fractures of the thigh illustrated by cases and a drawing. *Transactions of the New York Academy of Medicine*, **2**, 232.

FISK, G. R. (1944) The fractured femoral shaft: new approach to the problem. *Lancet*, **i**, 659.

JONES, A. R. (1953) John Haddy James. *Journal of Bone and Joint Surgery*, **35-B**, 661.

LIDGE, R. T. (1959) Complications following Bryant's traction in American Medical Association, section on Orthopaedic Surgery, Annual Meeting 1959. *Journal of Bone and Joint Surgery*, **41-A**, 1540.

MILLER, D. S., MARKIN, L. and GROSSMAN, E. (1952) Ischaemic fibrosis in lower extremity in children. *American Journal of Surgery*, **84**, 317.

NANGLE, E. J. (1951) *Instruments and Apparatus in Orthopaedic Surgery*, p. 9. Oxford: Blackwell.

NICHOLSON, J. T., FOSTER, R. M. and HEATH, R. D. (1955) Bryant's traction, a provocative cause of circulatory complications. *Journal of the American Medical Association*, **157**, 415.

NISSEN, K. (1971) Personal communication.

RUSSELL, R. H. (1924) Fractures of the femur: a clinical study. *British Journal of Surgery*, **11**, 491.

STRANGE, F. G. St. C. (1972) Personal communication.

THOMSON, S. A. and MAHONEY, L. J. (1951) Volkmann's ischaemic contracture and its relationship to fractures of the femur. *Journal of Bone and Joint Surgery*, **33-B**, 336.

5. Suspension of appliances

One initial difficulty in understanding traction is the presence of the many cords attached to both the patient and the appliance. The problem is simplified if it is recognised that the cords perform two distinct and separate functions: traction, described in Chapters 1, 3 and 4, and suspension of the appliance. (In the illustrations, *black* is used for suspension cords, and *red* for traction cords.)

By suspending appliances the mobility of the patient is increased, nursing is easier and the dangers of immobility—thrombosis and embolism, pressure sores, muscle wasting, joint stiffness and contractures, pneumonia, decalcification, renal stones and urinary infection—are decreased.

The appliance is suspended from an overhead frame by a series of counter-weights attached to it by cords which run over pulleys. A Thomas's splint can also be suspended by springs. The overhead frame is generally referred to as a Balkan beam, although each manufacturer uses a different name for his own overhead frame.

THE BALKAN BEAM

Overhead wooden beams were introduced during the Balkan Wars by a Dutch ambulance unit in 1903 (Bick, 1948). Today the Balkan beam is made from metal tubing which may be of round, square or octagonal cross section, depending upon the manufacturer. The methods of fixing the tubing to the bed differ, but the basic principle is the same.

Two uprights, one attached to each end of the bed, are joined by a longitudinal horizontal bar. Other shorter transverse horizontal bars may be attached to the uprights and to the longitudinal horizontal bar.

When a single Thomas's splint is to be suspended, only a single Balkan beam is required. One upright is attached to the centre of the top of the bed, and the other upright is attached to the same side of the foot of the bed as that on which the injured limb lies. If two splints or a plaster bed are to be suspended, two Balkan beams are required. The Balkan beams are attached to each side of the ends of the bed, and are joined together by the transverse horizontal bars.

SUSPENSION CORDS

Sash cord generally is used to suspend appliances. Easier recognition of the function of each cord in a traction-suspension system is possible if cords of two different colours are used, for example, red or green for traction cords, and white for suspension cords.

The cords must be attached firmly to the appliance. If they slip, the efficiency of the system is reduced and the patient may be injured. Many of the remarks made below apply also to the attachment of traction cords.

KNOTS

CLOVE HITCH (Fig. 5.1). A clove hitch is the best knot to use to attach a cord to an appliance, as it is self tightening and therefore is less likely to slip. It can be reinforced if necessary with a half hitch.

BARREL HITCH (Fig. 5.1). A barrel hitch is used to attach a single cord to a loop of cord. The position of the knot on the cord can be altered easily, by sliding the knot along the loop. When the correct position is obtained, the barrel hitch is converted to a reef knot as shown in Figure 5.2.

REEF KNOT (Fig. 5.1). The cords used in traction-suspension systems should not be joined, as the knots may jam in the pulleys. If it should be necessary to join two lengths of cord, a reef knot is used.

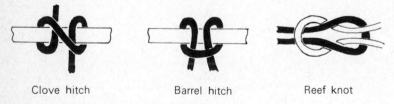

Clove hitch   Barrel hitch   Reef knot

Figure 5.1   Clove hitch, barrel hitch and reef knot.

After a knot is tied, the cord is cut about 2 inches (5·0 cm) away from the knot. The free end is bound to the main cord with a short length of zinc oxide strapping. This further reinforces the attachment of the cord to the appliance.

Even a clove hitch may slip on the side bars of a Thomas's splint. This can be prevented by wrapping a short length of zinc oxide strapping around the side bars over which the knot is tied.

The attachment of the cord to a Thomas's splint can be simplified and time saved by using short loops of linen tape. These loops are tied to the side bars of the Thomas's splint in the manner

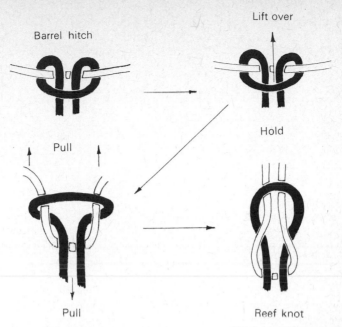

Figure 5.2   How to convert a barrel hitch into a reef knot.

of a barrel hitch (Fig. 5.1). The cords, attached to spring clips similar to those on a dog's lead, are clipped into the tape loops (Strange, 1972). Spring clips may be used to attach the cords to the weights.

PULLEYS

The function of a pulley is to control the direction of action of the weight attached to the end of the cord passing over the pulley. By altering the site of attachment of the cord and the pulley, or by using more than one pulley in the system, the force exerted by a given weight can be increased. This is termed the mechanical advantage of the system.

Large pulley wheels of 2 to $2\frac{1}{2}$ inches (5·0 to 6·25 cm) diameter and with $\frac{1}{4}$ inch (6 mm) diameter axles are preferable. Small rough cast pulley wheels, such as used for clothes lines, are less efficient. The majority of pulley wheels supplied by the manufacturers of orthopaedic supplies are made from Tuffnil, nylon or a similar synthetic material. All pulleys must be kept clean and oiled where necessary.

A compound pulley block (Fig. 5.3) consists of four small wheels on a common axle and one large wheel on its own axle, all enclosed in a common frame. The frame can be opened at one side to allow

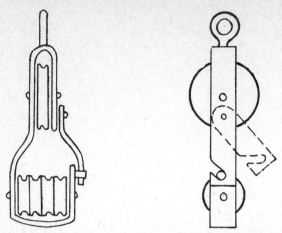

Figure 5.3   A compound pulley block, used in suspension of Thomas's splint (Fig. 5.7) and plaster bed (Fig. 5.11).

the cords to be slipped on and off the wheels. The cords attached to the appliance usually are looped over the smaller wheels, but if a pulley system with an increased mechanical advantage is required, the compound pulley block can be inverted. This arrangement is used in suspending a plaster bed (see page 50).

When suspending a Thomas's splint, the pulleys must be positioned correctly as the directions in which the cords run from the splint to the pulleys are important. The cords by their direction of pull keep the ring of the splint around the root of the limb, raise the splint off the mattress and thus enable the patient to move freely, and at the same time maintain the splint and thus the distal fragment of the fracture in correct alignment with the proximal fragment (Fig. 5.4).

CONTROL OF ROTATION

Rotation of the Thomas's splint around its long axis must be controlled, to prevent the limb from slipping off the splint and to prevent union of the fracture occurring in mal-rotation. Rotation is most likely to occur in a lateral direction.

The methods employed to control rotation are described below.

SUSPENSION WEIGHTS

The amount of weight required to suspend an appliance depends upon the weight of the appliance, the weight of the part of the

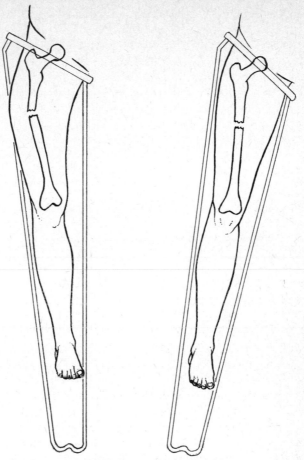

Figure 5.4 The distal fragment must be reduced to the proximal fragment. With a fracture at the junction of the middle and upper thirds of the femur, the proximal fragment is abducted as well as flexed, while the distal fragment is adducted. The splint, carrying the distal fragment, must therefore be abducted, otherwise there will be a varus deformity at the fracture site.

body suspended in the appliance, the mechanical advantage of the system employed for suspension, and the amount of friction present in the system.

The actual amount of weight required is determined by observing the behaviour of the suspension system. When the correct amount of weight is obtained, the appliance will move readily in all directions with little effort on the part of the patient, will return quickly to the position of rest, and will maintain the appliance in its correct relationship to the patient.

METHODS OF SUSPENDING A THOMAS'S SPLINT

Fracture boards are placed under the mattress to ensure a firm base.

A suspended Thomas's splint is entirely free from the bed, except at its upper end where the back of the padded ring rests on the mattress. The patient can raise his pelvis off the bed by pulling up with his arms on a patient's helper, aided by downward pressure on the bed with his other foot. The whole of the injured limb, from the ischial tuberosity to the foot, moves in one piece with the patient's trunk, and therefore the position of the fracture is unchanged.

Using cords, pulleys and weights

A Thomas's splint may be suspended in a number of different ways using cords, pulleys and weights. The details differ but the principles are the same.

1. The cords must be attached firmly to the splint. Different methods of attaching the cords to the splint have been described above.
2. The Thomas's splint must not move independently of the lower limb. In fixed traction the counter-traction force is directed up the side bars of the splint (Fig. 3.1), and therefore the ring of the splint remains around the root of the limb. In sliding traction, counter-traction is obtained by raising the foot of the bed to utilize body weight. The splint only supports the limb. If a cranially-directed force is not applied to the splint, the splint may be pulled down the limb with serious consequences for the position of the fracture.
3. The pulleys must be positioned correctly and run smoothly.
4. Rotation of the Thomas's splint must be controlled.
5. The suspension weights must be adjusted carefully.

Method one (Fig. 5.5)
Small loops of cord are formed between the side bars of the splint at each end. The suspension cords are attached to the centre of each loop using a barrel hitch, and are then passed upwards and cranially to pulleys. From these pulleys the cords pass to other pulleys situated at the head or foot of the bed, before running vertically down to weights.

Rotation of the splint is adjusted by moving the position of the knots on the proximal and distal loops, until the correct position is obtained, when the barrel hitches are converted to reef knots.

The disadvantages of this system are that the proximal cord

passes close to the patient's face, the ring of the splint is not adequately retained in the groin, and the patient's mobility is limited.

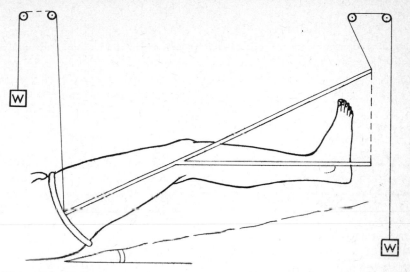

Figure 5.5 Method 1. Suspension of Thomas's splint. Separate suspension cords and weights are attached to each end of the Thomas's splint.

Method two (Fig. 5.6)

Two lengths of cord, one on each side, are attached to each end of the splint. Each cord passes over two pulleys. A suspension weight is attached firmly to both cords at a point nearer the pelvis.

Rotation is controlled by adjusting the length of each cord. By shortening the outer cord slightly, medial rotation of the splint is obtained.

The disadvantages of this system are that the suspension weight is directly over the patient's thigh and, unless it is attached firmly to the cords, it may fall injuring the patient, and the mobility of the patient is limited.

This system of suspension is satisfactory for the suspension of a Thomas's splint when fixed traction is used.

Method three (Fig. 5.7)

Dommisse and Nangle (1947) described a method of suspending a Thomas's splint using a compound pulley block.

Two lengths of cord, one on each side, are attached to each end of the splint. These cords must not be too long. Both cords pass over the smaller wheels of a compound pulley block, situated over the patient's thigh. A cord passes up from the ring above the larger wheel, over a pulley attached to the overhead frame, down and round the larger wheel of the compound pulley block and then up

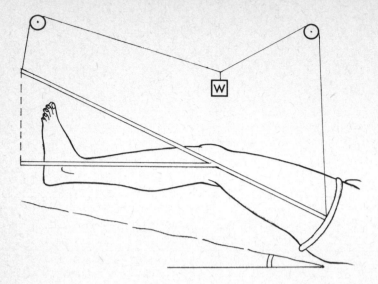

Figure 5.6   Method 2. Suspension of Thomas's splint. Two cords pass on each side from top to bottom of the Thomas's splint. The suspension weight is firmly attached to both cords, more towards the pelvis.

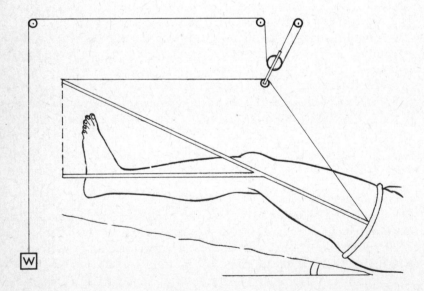

Figure 5.7   Method 3. Suspension of Thomas's splint. A compound pulley block (Fig 5.3) is used. Two cords pass from top to bottom of the splint, one on each side, passing over the smaller wheels of the compound pulley block.

again and round a second pulley before passing towards the foot of the bed. There the cord passes over another pulley before running vertically down to a weight. The arrangement of the pulleys and cords produces a suspension system with a mechanical advantage of three to one. A suspension weight of 8 lb (3·6 kg) is usually adequate.

In this arrangement the splint pivots around the smaller wheels of the compound pulley block, the height of which can vary. If the proximal end of the splint is raised and the distal end lowered, the pulley block moves proximally, and the force directed cranially is increased, thus preventing the splint from slipping down the leg.

If the front of the ring of the splint presses upon the patient's thigh, the pulleys attached to the overhead frame are moved cranially.

Rotation of the splint is controlled by varying the length of the cords attached to each end of the splint. Further fine adjustment is obtained by varying the position of the cords on the smaller wheels of the pulley block.

This is an excellent system of suspension and it can be used with either fixed or sliding traction.

Method four

Setting up the suspension systems described above takes time. The time taken can be reduced considerably if a bed with an overhead frame, pulleys, cords and weights is prepared beforehand.

Strange (1972) utilizes such an arrangement with sliding traction with a 'fixed' Thomas's splint. The overhead frame (Thanet beam— Fig. 5.8) consists of one vertical upright attached to the centre of the head of the bed, and two vertical uprights attached to each side of the foot of the bed. These uprights are joined by two longitudinal horizontal bars. From a short transverse horizontal bar attached to the top of the single upright at the head of the bed, eight pulleys are suspended, four for each lower limb on each side of the upright (Fig. 5.8a). Four pulleys are attached to each longitudinal horizontal bar, two each at the level of the hip and the foot (Fig. 5.8b and 5.8c). A second transverse horizontal bar carrying two pulleys for the traction cords, joins the two uprights at the foot of the bed (Fig. 5.8c).

Eight cords with spring clips attached to each end are threaded through each of the eight pulleys suspended from the transverse bar at the head of the bed. Weights, which hang down behind the head of the bed, are attached to one end of each cord (Fig. 5.8a). The bed is thus ready to receive a patient.

Four suspension cords which must be at right angles to the splint are attached by the spring clips to loops of tape placed around the side bars of the Thomas's splint. The proximal loops are situated at the padded ring and the distal loops level with the foot. The

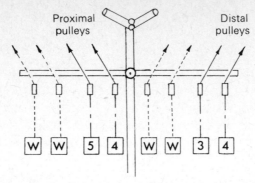

Figure 5.8a   Thanet beam. Arrangement of pulleys, cords and weights on horizontal transverse bar at the head of the bed (weights in lbs).

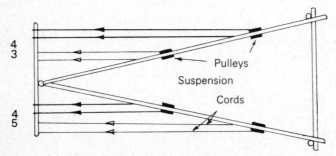

Figure 5.8b   Thanet beam. Plan view.

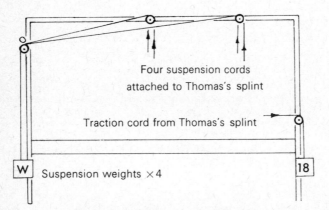

Figure 5.8c   Thanet beam. Side view.

Figure 5.8   Thanet beam: pulleys, cords and weights.

weights attached to the two cords from the outer side bar of the splint are one pound (0·45 kg) heavier than those attached to the corresponding cords from the inner side bar (Fig. 5.9). In this way lateral rotation of the splint is controlled. Listed below are the suspension weights commonly used for adults. They have to be modified only rarely.

5.0 lb. (2.3 kg)   4.0 lb. (1.8 kg)

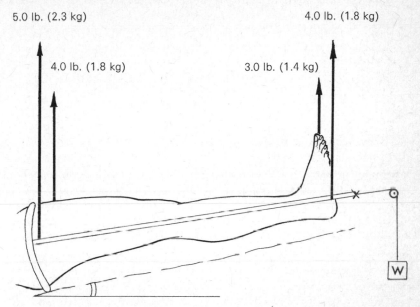

4.0 lb. (1.8 kg)   3.0 lb. (1.4 kg)

Figure 5.9   Method 4. Suspension of Thomas's splint. Arrangement of suspension weights for sliding traction in a 'fixed' Thomas's splint, using a Thanet beam (Strange, 1972).

> Proximal end of splint, outer side bar—5 lb (2·3 kg)
> inner side bar—4 lb (1·8 kg)
> Distal end of splint,   outer side bar—4 lb (1·8 kg)
> inner side bar—3 lb (1·4 kg)

As sliding traction with a 'fixed' Thomas's splint is employed with this system of suspension, the suspension cords only have to suspend the splint; they do not have to maintain the position of the splint on the limb. The patient rapidly becomes very mobile, so mobile in fact that within two to three weeks of injury he is able to climb onto the overhead frame or stand by the side of his bed on his sound limb without any displacement of the fracture occurring.

Using springs

A Thomas's splint, to which a Böhler stirrup has been attached by brackets* at the centre of gravity of the limb near the knee, can be suspended from an overhead frame by a single spring incorporating

---

* See Appendix.

a safety cord, and with a hook at each end (Denman, 1962). The spring passes upwards and cranially from the Böhler stirrup to the overhead frame.

Springs, of three different tensions, which measure 18 inches (46·0 cm) in length when lax and which stretch 6 inches (15·0 cm) in response to pulls of 15, 20, and 25 lb (6·8, 9·0, and 11·3 kg) respectively, are available.* Usually the spring of intermediate tension is used.

Rotation is controlled by varying the attachment of the spring to the Böhler stirrup.

SUSPENSION OF THE FISK SPLINT (Fisk, 1944)

The Fisk splint (see Chapters 2 and 4) is suspended from three points on an overhead beam. The end of the knee-flexion piece is suspended by a single cord looped over the overhead beam. The length of this cord is such that when the hip is flexed to an angle of 45 degrees, the leg is horizontal. The ends of a second long loop of cord are attached to the eyelets at the corners of the squared-off frame. This second loop passes upwards and cranially over a pulley on the overhead beam, situated over the patient's abdomen. It is attached to a *single* suspension weight of usually 4 to 8 lb (1·8 to 3·6 kg) which is passed through the loop by a slip knot, and which hangs within easy reach of the patient. This suspension cord is at right angles to the long axis of the femur when the hip is flexed to an angle of 45 degrees (Fig. 5.10).

The patient flexes his hip, assisting the movement by pulling down on the suspension weight, and at the same time flexes his knee and dorsiflexes his ankle. The patient then actively extends his hip and knee and plantar-flexes his ankle while gradually releasing his pull on the suspension weight. Passive movements are not encouraged.

Rotation is controlled by varying the length of each attachment of the fixed cord to the end of the knee-flexion piece, and by varying the tension in the loop of cord attached to the squared-off frame.

SUSPENSION OF TULLOCH BROWN TIBIAL U-LOOP

The Tulloch Brown tibial U-loop can be suspended either by using the same arrangement of cord, pulleys and one weight as employed

* See Appendix.

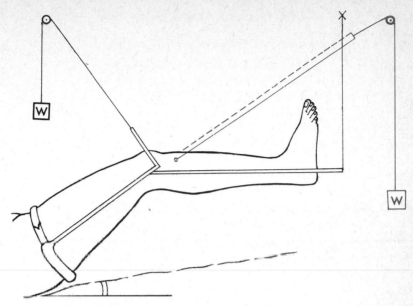

Figure 5.10   Suspension of the Fisk splint.

in Russell traction (Fig. 4.4), or by using a simple pulley system and two weights as illustrated in Figure 4.6.

Rotation is controlled by varying the site of attachment of the cord to the Nissen stirrup.

PREVENTION OF EQUINUS DEFORMITY AT THE ANKLE

When a lower limb is immobilised in recumbency for any length of time, weakness of the muscles of dorsiflexion of the ankle may occur with subsequent contraction of the posterior capsule of the ankle joint and the development of fixed equinus deformity at the ankle.

To reduce the risk of this occurring, active dorsiflexion of the ankle must be commenced immediately and be carried out regularly. The risk can be reduced further by providing a support for the foot. This can be achieved in several ways.

1. *A foot piece*, a U-shaped length of metal which is clamped to the side bars of the Thomas's splint level with the sole of the foot. The foot rests upon a sling which passes between the limbs of the U-loop.
2. *Stockinette*. A length of stockinette, knotted at one end, is pulled over the foot like a sock. A cord, tied to the knotted end of the stockinette is passed cranially over a pulley to a small weight.

3. *Traction unit.* In a traction unit the foot is supported by the plaster cast.
4. *Nissen foot plate* in U-loop tibial pin traction and suspension.
5. When a Fisk splint is used, a long length of elastic can be tied to the eyelets of the squared-off frame and passed round the sole of a slipper to which it is stitched.

SUSPENSION OF A PLASTER BED

Dommisse and Nangle (1947) and Nangle (1951) described a method by which a plaster bed may be suspended, using compound pulleys.

Two overhead frames joined together by transverse bars are required. The transverse bar at the level of the shoulders must be 12 inches (30·0 cm) longer than the one at the level of the knees, to give the suspension cords a clear run and to prevent the weights from fouling each other.

The plaster shell is attached to a wooden frame provided with two cross bars. One cross bar is situated just below the shoulders and the other level with the knees. The shoulder bar must be long enough to prevent the suspension cords from rubbing on the patient's arms.

A compound pulley is inverted and attached to each end of the shoulder and knee bars of the wooden frame. Two single pulleys are attached on each side at each level to the transverse horizontal bars of the overhead frames. The arrangement of the cords and pulleys is illustrated in Figure 5.11. The mechanical advantage in the shoulder and knee systems is four to one and three to one respectively.

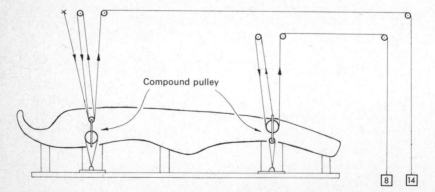

Figure 5.11 Arrangement of cords for suspension of a plaster bed. Note: Arrows show direction in which cords run. The compound pulleys are attached to the wooden frame which supports the plaster bed, in opposite directions at the shoulders and knees.

The amount of weight required is determined for each patient. An average adult requires two 14 lb (6·3 kg) weights for the shoulder system and two 8 lb (3·6 kg) weights for the knee system. The effect of these weights multiplied by the mechanical advantage (M.A.) of the pulley systems is as follows:

Shoulder bar system $2 \times (14\,lb \times 4) = 112\,lb\,(50·4\,kg)$
Knee bar system $2 \times (\ 8\,lb \times 3) = \ \ 48\,lb\,(21·6\,kg)$

                             Total lift $= 160\,lb\,(72·0\,kg)$

The counter-weights must be heavy enough to enable the patient and the plaster bed to be raised easily from the bed and to remain suspended.

SUSPENSION OF A PELVIC SLING

Minor pelvic fractures, for example isolated fractures of the pubic or ischial rami, are treated by rest in bed. When the pelvic ring has been opened out, a pelvic sling is used (Fig. 5.12). A pelvic sling

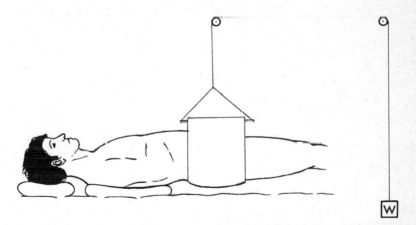

Figure 5.12 Pelvic sling. The pelvic sling lies between the symphysis pubis and the posterior iliac crests. Sufficient weights are used to just lift the buttocks off the bed. There are pillows under the back and the head. The suspension cords are crossed if inward pressure is required.

is made from heavy canvas or Terylene 12 inches (30·0 cm) wide. It has hems at each side through which large diameter wooden or steel rods are passed. Cords pass from the pelvic sling over pulleys to weights.

APPLICATION OF A PELVIC SLING

- Place the pelvic sling under the buttocks, to lie between the symphysis pubis and the posterior iliac crests.
- Attach a cord to each end of the rods.
- Pass the cords over pulleys situated above the pelvic sling, and attach sufficient weights to lift the patient's buttocks just clear of the mattress.
- Place pillows under the patient's shoulders and back, to keep the patient horizontal and to avoid the sling's slipping up or down.
- To close the pelvic ring, cross the suspension cords to produce an inward pressure.
- Combine a pelvic sling with skeletal limb traction when there is upward displacement of one side of the pelvis.

REFERENCES

BICK, E. M. (1948) *Source Book of Orthopaedics*, p. 284. Baltimore: Williams & Wilkins.

DENMAN, E. E. (1962) Spring suspension for Thomas's splint. *British Medical Journal*, **ii**, 47.

DOMMISSE, G. F. and NANGLE, E. J. (1947) The elimination of apparatus inertia in the treatment of fractures. *British Journal of Surgery*, **34**, 395.

FISK, G. R. (1944) The fractured femoral shaft: new approach to the problem. *Lancet*, **i**, 659.

NANGLE, E. J. (1951) *Instruments and Apparatus in Orthopaedic Surgery*, p. 89. Oxford: Blackwell.

STRANGE, F. G. St. C. (1972) Personal communication.

6. The management of patients in traction

The correct management of patients in traction is very important if good results are to be obtained with this method of treatment. *Patients in traction and traction-suspension systems do not look after themselves.*

Daily checks must be made to ensure that complications are not occurring and that the traction and suspension systems are working efficiently. Regular radiological examinations of the position of the fracture and the correct interpretation of these radiographs are necessary. Physiotherapy to the whole patient, as well as to the injured part, is vital to ensure that when the fracture has united the general condition of the patient and the condition of the injured limb are such that full function is regained as quickly as possible. Lastly, at some stage the decision to discard splintage completely must be taken.

THE PATIENT

Every patient in traction must be questioned *daily*, and the limb or limbs in traction examined *daily* for the presence or absence of the following:

PAIN. Pain may result from pressure sores developing in the groin, around the ankle, under the strapping or over the sacrum. In children who are being managed in modified Bryant's traction for congenital dislocation of the hip, pain may result from impingement of the femoral head on the superior lip of the acetabulum.

PARAESTHESIA OR NUMBNESS in the injured limb. This may result from the impairment of normal nerve function by ischaemia, pressure or excessive traction upon a nerve.

SKIN IRRITATION from allergy to adhesive strapping.

THE PRESENCE OF SWELLING from having applied the bandage too tightly, venous thrombosis or lack of exercise.

THE POWER OF ANKLE AND TOE MOVEMENTS. The power of these movements may be reduced as a result of impairment of nerve function, disuse and muscular atrophy.

THE ACTIVE AND PASSIVE MOVEMENT OF THE ANKLES AND TOES, and of the other joints of the body. Reduced dorsiflexion of the ankle joint from contraction of the calf muscles and the posterior capsule of the joint may occur if the foot is allowed to lie in plantarflexion.

Painful limitation of dorsiflexion of the hallux suggests ischaemia of the flexor hallucis longus muscle; that of the fingers, ischaemia of the deep flexor muscles of the forearm.

THE PRESENCE OR ABSENCE OF THE PERIPHERAL PULSES, and the colour and temperature of the fingers and toes. It must be remembered that the circulation in muscles can be impaired even although the peripheral pulses are palpable.

THE TRACTION-SUSPENSION SYSTEM

The traction-suspension system must be checked *daily*, and after each period of physiotherapy or radiological examination.

THE POSITION OF THE SPLINT. The splint must fit snugly around the root of the limb and must be abducted, adducted or flexed sufficiently to maintain the correct alignment of the distal fragment of the fracture with the proximal fragment.

THE BANDAGES may be stained from an underlying pressure sore or skin excoriation. A loose bandage must be reapplied.

ADHESIVE STRAPPING must not be wrinkled or have slid down the limb.

THE STEINMANN PIN, etc, must be immobile in the bone. The skin wounds must be dry and not inflamed. If the skin wounds are moist or inflamed, or the pin is loose in the bone, infection of the pin track may be present or imminent. When a tibial pin track is infected, percussion over the tibial tuberosity is painful. When infection of the pin track is present, the pin must be removed as soon as possible, and an alternative method of traction substituted.

THE BÖHLER STIRRUP, if present, must move freely on the pin, otherwise movement of the stirrup will be imparted to the pin. A drop of sterile glycerine can be used for lubrication.

THE VARIOUS SLINGS must be positioned accurately and be at the correct tension. Movement of the slings on the side bars of the splint can be prevented by wrapping a few turns of strapping around the side bars before fitting the slings.

PADS if used must be of the correct thickness and must be sited correctly.

THE TRACTION AND SUSPENSION CORDS must be on the pulleys and be able to move freely. They must not be frayed.

THE TRACTION AND SUSPENSION WEIGHTS must be off the floor and must hang free of the bed.

THE END OF THE BED must be elevated to provide counter-traction in the opposite direction to the traction force, when sliding traction is used.

RADIOLOGICAL EXAMINATION

When a fracture is managed in either fixed or sliding traction, regular radiological control with two exposures taken at right angles to each other is essential throughout the period of immobilisation, to ensure that reduction of the fracture is achieved and maintained until union occurs. A rough guide to the frequency of radiological examination is:

Twice in the first week, then
Once a week for the next three weeks, then
Once a month until union occurs.
After each manipulation of the fracture.
After each change in the traction weight.

PHYSIOTHERAPY

Hugh Owen Thomas (1876) emphasised the 'combination of enforced, uninterrupted and prolonged rest; the first gives relief from pain, the second, added to the first, enables the case steadily to progress to a cure, the third secures that which has been gained', whereas Lucas-Championnière (1895) believed that the full function of a limb returned earlier if muscle and joint contractures were prevented. The correct management of a fracture depends upon obtaining a balance between these two concepts so that the fracture unites in the best functional position as rapidly as possible, the development of joint stiffness is prevented or minimised, as much muscle power as possible is retained, demineralisation of the skeleton is minimal, and the risk of pneumonia, venous thrombosis and renal calculi is decreased (British Orthopaedic Association, 1955).

The mental and physical condition of the whole patient as well as the condition of the injured limb is very important. Rehabilitation is begun immediately, its intensity increasing as union of the fracture progresses, becoming maximal when union has occurred.

The traction-suspension system employed in the management of a fracture should allow as much activity of the patient as possible, consistent with the requirements of the fracture itself. Every patient must be encouraged repeatedly to be as active as possible. Many patients being treated in traction-suspension systems are afraid that they will upset the system or the reduction of the fracture if they move. It must be emphasised that this will not occur. If it does, the fault is that of the doctor who set up the system, and not that of the patient.

In addition to encouraging the patient to be as active as possible, supervised physiotherapy is essential throughout the period of immobilisation.

Although some traction-suspension systems used in the management of fractures of the femoral shaft limit the possible range of knee movement or the general mobility of the patient more than others, the following general management is advised.

Immediately instruct the patient to carry out for ten minutes every hour :

Quadriceps exercises.

As much active flexion and extension of the knee as the system allows.

Active dorsiflexion and plantarflexion of the ankle.

Active inversion and eversion of the foot.

When the fracture is clinically firm (usually 6 to 8 weeks for a fracture of the femoral shaft) *commence, out of traction and under supervision,* daily assisted knee flexion and extension exercises, and straight-leg raising. If pain at the fracture site develops, delay this treatment until the fracture is more soundly united. Care must be taken that the traction-suspension system is adjusted correctly after treatment.

If fixed traction in a Thomas's splint is used, reduce the amount of knee flexion in traction to 5 to 10 degrees. This will assist in the recovery of quadriceps power.

When sliding traction in a Fisk splint, or in a Thomas's splint with an individually suspended knee-flexion piece, is employed, the range of knee movement possible is greater than with other systems.

WHEN TO DISCARD THE SPLINT

When a fracture of the femoral shaft is treated conservatively, it is difficult to decide when splintage can be discarded completely. It is essentially a compromise between discarding the splint as early as possible to allow maximal rehabilitation of the patient and the injured limb, and not so early that complications occur at the fracture site. The dangers of discarding the splint too early are late angulation at the fracture site and refracture of the femur.

Do not discard the splint completely if—

1. Movement at the fracture site is present.
2. There is definite tenderness of the callus.
3. Radiographs show—
    (a) Only a small amount of callus to be present.
    (b) The callus to be located mainly on one side of the fracture.
    (c) The presence of fine cracks in the cortex of one or other of the major fragments (Seimon, 1964).
4. There is a tendency to late angulation.

Charnley (1970) stated that the occurrence of late angulation or spontaneous refracture of the femur is preceded by a decrease in the range of knee flexion. He suggested that there should be a minimum period of twelve weeks in splintage. After twelve weeks the range of knee movement should be measured daily during an initial trial period of one week without splintage. If during this time there has not been a decrease in the range of knee movement, late angulation or spontaneous refracture of the femur is unlikely, and therefore the splint can be discarded completely.

REFERENCES

BRITISH ORTHOPAEDIC ASSOCIATION (1955) Debate on 'That Lucas-Championnière was right'. British Orthopaedic Association Meeting, Liverpool, October 7, 1955. *Journal of Bone and Joint Surgery*, **37-B**, 719.

CHARNLEY, J. (1970) *The Closed Treatment of Common Fractures*. 3rd ed., p. 189. Edinburgh and London: Churchill Livingstone.

LUCAS-CHAMPIONNIÈRE, J. (1895) *Traitement des Fractures par le Massage et la Mobilisation*. Paris. Rueff et Cie.

SEIMON, L. P. (1964) Refracture of the shaft of the femur. *Journal of Bone and Joint Surgery*, **46-B**, 32.

THOMAS, H. O. (1876) *Diseases of the Hip, Knee and Ankle Joints, with Their Deformities, Treated by a New and Efficient Method*, 2nd ed., p. iii. Liverpool: T. Dobb & Co.

7. Spinal traction

In the management of conditions of the cervical spine, traction may be obtained by applying apparatus around the head (non-skeletal or halter traction) or to the skull (skeletal or skull traction). A cord passes from the apparatus over a pulley, attached to the head of the bed, to a traction weight. In an ambulant patient, fixed skeletal traction to the cervical spine can be obtained by using the halo traction method.

When traction is required for correction of deformities of the thoracic and lumbar spines, skeletal traction using the halo-pelvic method is employed. Halo and halo-pelvic traction will be discussed separately.

NON-SKELETAL OR HALTER TRACTION

Halter traction is uncomfortable if it is applied continuously for more than a few hours. It is reserved usually for use in the treatment of cervical spondylosis as an out-patient.

A canvas or chamois leather head halter may be used (Fig. 7.1).

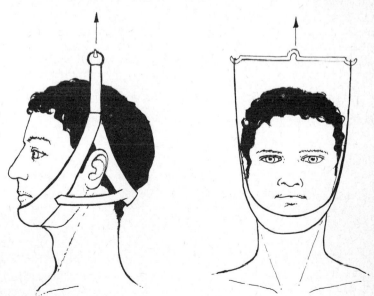

Figure 7.1 Canvas head halter.

One part is placed under the chin and the other under the occiput. A metal spreader hooks onto the two side pieces to avoid lateral compression of the soft tissues when traction is applied. A cord from the metal spreader passes over a pulley fixed to the top of the bed and is attached to weights. The maximum weight which can be attached is 3 to 5 lb (1·4 to 2·3 kg). Pressure sores may develop under the chin or occiput, and in men beard growth may be troublesome. Eating is difficult. **The Crile head halter** (Fig. 7.2) consists of a well-padded curved metal bar, resembling a horse collar, which is placed under the occiput. A padded forehead piece is attached by straps to the occipital piece. The chin is free. The maximum weight which can be attached is 3 to 5 lb (1·4 to 2·3 kg).

The head of the bed must be raised to provide counter-traction.

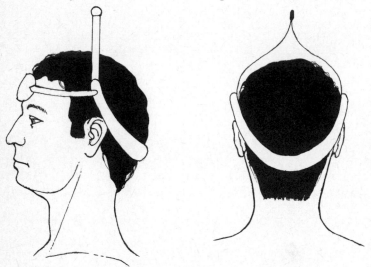

Figure 7.2 Crile head halter.

SKELETAL OR SKULL TRACTION

Skeletal or skull traction (Crutchfield, 1933) is achieved by gaining a purchase on the outer table of the skull with metal pins. Crutchfield or Cone (Barton) tongs may be used. A traction weight of 20 to 40 lb (9·1 to 18·2 kg) can be applied.

Skull traction is used commonly in the management of serious injuries to the cervical spine to reduce a dislocation or fracture-dislocation. In traction, the fracture or fracture-dislocation is under control and injury to the spinal cord is less likely to occur. Skull traction is used also to maintain the position of the cervical spine before and after operative fusion and for the treatment of cervical spondylosis with severe nerve root compression symptoms.

Crutchfield tongs

Crutchfield tongs (Fig. 7.3) fit into the parietal bones. A special drill point with a shoulder is used to enable an accurate depth of hole to be drilled (Crutchfield, 1954).

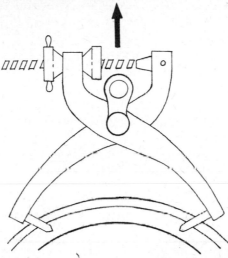

Figure 7.3 Crutchfield tongs. Note that the points of the tongs are almost at right angles to the line of traction.

APPLICATION OF CRUTCHFIELD TONGS
- Sedate the patient.
- Shave the scalp locally. Excessive shaving is very distressing to the patient.
- Draw a line on the scalp, bisecting the skull from front to back (Fig. 7.4).

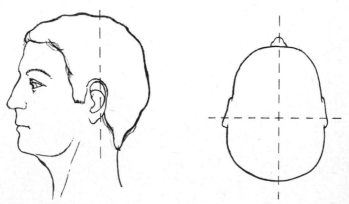

Figure 7.4 Skull markings for positioning Cruthfield tongs. A vertical line through the tips of the mastoid processes crosses at right angles a second line bisecting the skull from front to back.

- Draw a second line joining the tips of the mastoid processes (the plane of the cervical articulations) which crosses the first line at right angles (Fig. 7.4).
- Fully open out the tongs.
- With the fully open tongs lying equally on each side of the antero-posterior line, press the points into the scalp making dimples on the second line.
- Infiltrate the area of the dimples down to and including the periosteum, with local anaesthetic solution.
- Make small stab wounds in the scalp at the dimples.
- Using the special drill point, drill through the outer table of the skull *in a direction parallel to the points of the tongs.* The drill point is inserted to a depth of 3 millimetres in children, care being taken because of the scanty diploic space, and 4 millimetres in adults.
- Fit the points of the tongs into the drill holes.
- Tighten the adjustment screw until a firm grip is obtained, *and repeat daily for the first 3 to 4 days,* and then tighten when necessary.
- Attach a traction cord to the two lugs.
- Attach a weight to the traction cord (see page 64).
- Raise the head of the bed to provide counter-traction. Elevation must be increased as the traction weight is increased.

Failure of the procedure

Crutchfield (1954) stated that failure may be due to several factors.

1. The use of a faulty instrument. When opened out fully, the distance between the points should be 11 cm and certainly not less than 10 cm.
2. The pins must be long enough to prevent the arms of the tongs from crushing the scalp, and they must be set obliquely enough to ensure that they penetrate the diploe almost at right angles to the line of traction.
3. Placing the drill holes too close together in the skull.
4. Insufficient penetration of the skull.
5. Failure to keep the tongs tight.

Cone (Barton) tongs

The tongs were designed by Barton (Cone and Turner, 1937). A drill is not required for their insertion (Fig. 7.5). The threaded steel points are screwed into the parietal bones behind the ears.

APPLICATION OF CONE (BARTON) TONGS
- Sedate the patient.
- Draw a line up from the tip of the mastoid process to cross the sagittal plane at right angles (Fig. 7.6).
- Shave the skull above and behind the ears.
- Open out the tongs sufficiently, and determine where the conical ends lie on the line drawn above.

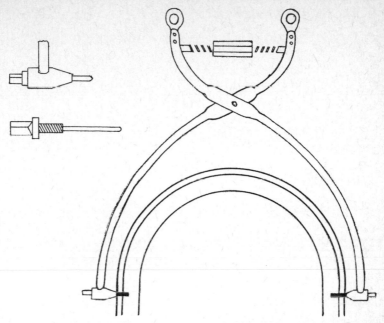

Figure 7.5 Cone (Barton) tongs. No separate drilling is required. The special steel points are inserted into the conical ends of the tongs and tightened alternately.

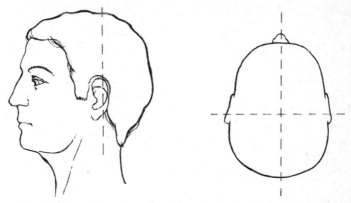

Figure 7.6 Skull markings for Cone tongs. A vertical line through the mastoid process crosses at right angles a second line bisecting the skull from front to back.

- Infiltrate this area with local anaesthetic solution.
- Reapply the tongs with the conical ends pressed firmly against the scalp.
- Insert both steel points into the conical ends and tighten each one alternately, driving the points through the outer table of the skull.
- Attach a traction cord to the two lugs.
- Attach a weight to the traction cord (see page 64).
- Elevate the head of the bed to provide counter-traction. Elevation must be increased as the traction weight is increased.

Management of skull traction

Dislocation or fracture-dislocation of the cervical spine

The majority of serious injuries to the cervical spine result from forward flexion with or without an element of lateral flexion, and are therefore relatively stable in extension. Occasionally extension injuries occur, in which cases the spine is stable in flexion. In all injuries, rotation of the spine is dangerous.

It is not advisable to attempt a rapid reduction of a dislocation or fracture-dislocation of the cervical spine, as the spinal cord may be damaged if the initial pull is excessive.

Aims of treatment

1. To avoid damage to the cervical cord.
2. To restore the antero-posterior diameter of the spinal canal.
3. To obtain complete reduction of the dislocation or fracture-dislocation. Although this is desirable it is not always possible. A decrease in the antero-posterior diameter of the spinal canal of less than 3 mm may be accepted (Rogers, 1957).

PROCEDURE

● Apply tongs as described above.
● Apply minimum traction weight (see below).
● Take radiographs the following day.
● If reduction has not been obtained, gradually increase the traction weight. It is rarely necessary to more than double the minimum traction weight.
● When sufficient distraction has been obtained—
  1. Do not increase the traction weight further.
  2. Extend the cervical spine by placing a small rolled towel or sand-bag *under the neck* (*not* under the head as this will flex the cervical spine).
● When satisfactory alignment has been obtained, reduce the traction weight to 5 to 7 lb (2·3 to 3·2 kg) to maintain the corrected position, until the spine is stable. This takes 6 to 10 weeks.
● If a heavy traction weight is used initially, take radiographs at 15 minute intervals for at least one hour, or until it can be seen that the traction force is not too strong, and reduce the traction weight as soon as sufficient distraction has been obtained.

Recommended traction weights,

for correction of deformity only (Crutchfield, 1954).

Level	Minimum weight	Maximum weight
C1	5 lb (2·3 kg)	10 lb (4·5 kg)
C2	6 lb (2·7 kg)	10 to 12 lb (4·5 to 5·4 kg)
C3	8 lb (3·6 kg)	10 to 15 lb (4·5 to 6·7 kg)
C4	10 lb (4·5 kg)	15 to 20 lb (6·7 to 9·0 kg)
C5	12 lb (5·4 kg)	20 to 25 lb (9·0 to 11·3 kg)
C6	15 lb (6·7 kg)	20 to 30 lb (9·0 to 13·5 kg)
C7	18 lb (8·2 kg)	25 to 35 lb (11·3 to 15·8 kg)

These traction weights are approximately correct for the various levels of the cervical spine when the head of the patient's bed is raised not more than 20 degrees for the purpose of counter traction.

Important: check daily that:
1. There has not been a change in the neurological examination of the patient.
2. The tongs are firmly applied to the skull. Tighten as necessary.
3. The scalp wounds are not infected.
4. The traction cord runs freely in the pulley and is not frayed.
5. The traction weight is hanging free.

Complications of skull traction

Skeletal traction applied to the skull may give rise to complications which may be fatal—osteomyelitis of the skull, extradural haematoma, extradural abscess, subdural abscess, cerebral abscess (Weisl, 1971).

These complications may be heralded by pyrexia and headaches, and progress to fits, hemiplegia and coma. Examination of the cerebrospinal fluid and cerebral angiography may be normal. In the presence of osteomyelitis of the skull, radiographic examination may show radiolucent areas at the site of insertion of the pins.

If infection is suspected, the scalp wounds must be swabbed to discover the infecting organism and its antibiotic sensitivity, and the tongs removed, another method of controlling the cervical spine being substituted.

Halo traction

The halo traction apparatus (Fig 7.7) consists of a jointed adjustable skull frame incorporated in a plaster jacket which extends from the shoulders to the iliac crests, the neck being free from plaster (Perry and Nickel, 1959). This is a method of applying fixed skeletal traction to the cervical spine, purchase on the body being obtained by the close moulding of the plaster jacket around the iliac crests. Patients in halo traction are ambulant.

Halo traction comprises:
1. A U-shaped metal bracket fixed to the shoulder straps of the plaster jacket.
2. Two angled vertical steel rods fitted into vertical sockets in the U-bracket.
3. An adjustable rectangular frame with three transverse bars (the anterior and middle bars carry the three supporting arms of the halo; the posterior bar gives rigidity) attached to the upper ends of the vertical rods.

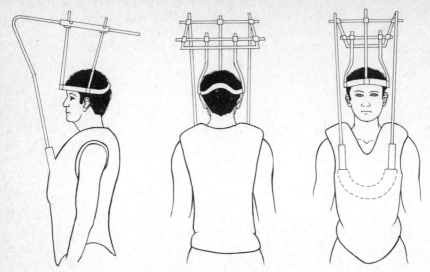

Figure 7.7   Halo traction.

4. The halo splint—an oval steel band arched upwards posteriorly to clear the occipital area, with four sets of three threaded holes at 2, 4, 8, and 10 o'clock. Four screws, one for each set of holes, are passed into the outer table of the skull. The screws have small sharp points which rapidly flare out onto broad shoulders, creating a large area of contact against the skull with the minimum of penetration.
5. Three supporting arms fix the halo splint to the rectangular frame. All the supporting arms can be adjusted in an antero-posterior direction by altering the position of the anterior and middle transverse bars. Lateral adjustment is by altering the position of the supporting arms on the transverse bars.

APPLICATION OF HALO TRACTION
The application of halo traction is carried out in two stages (Thompson, 1962; Nickel, *et al.*, 1968).
Application of the plaster jacket
● Fit Crutchfield tongs to control an unstable spine.
● Sit the patient on a stool with vertical traction on the Crutchfield tongs.
● Place 1½ inch (3·75 cm) thick sorbo-rubber or orthopaedic felt over the shoulders.
● Apply a plaster jacket from the shoulders down to the iliac crests, where it must be moulded accurately.
● Return the patient to his bed.
Fitting of the traction apparatus—48 hours later
● Choose a halo splint which is about ½ inch (1·25 cm) larger than the circumference of the patient's head. Autoclave the splint, screws and locking nuts.

- Lie the patient over the end of an operating table with the shoulder pieces of the jacket projecting over the end of the table.
- Maintain control of the cervical spine by manual traction.
- Shave the patient's head for a distance of about 2 inches (5·0 cm) around each screw site, and prepare the partly shaven scalp.
- Scrub up.
- Advance one screw in each quadrant about ½ inch (1·25 cm) through a selected screw hole—use the middle holes initially.
- Slip the halo splint over the skull and position it so that the lower margin of the splint lies just above the ears and about ¼ inch (6·0 mm) above the eyebrows.
- Mark the point of penetration of the skull on the scalp with Bonney's Blue, by sighting along the previously advanced screws. The anterior screws are inserted in the shallow grooves on the forehead between the supra-orbital ridges and the frontal protuberances.
- Remove the halo splint.
- Infiltrate each of the above marks with 2 to 3 ml of 2 per cent local anaesthetic solution.
- Slip the halo splint on again and advance all the screws until they touch the scalp at the previously marked points.
- Adjust the screws so that the halo splint lies symmetrically around the skull.
- Advance the screws using a torque-limiting screwdriver preset to 5·5 lb/inches (6·34 kg/cm) until slip occurs. The screws must be advanced *in diametrically opposed pairs at the same time*, to avoid side-to-side drifting of the halo splint. Incision of the scalp is not required. Tighten the locking nut on each screw.
- Assemble the steel superstructure.
- Fix the U-bracket to the plaster jacket with plaster.
- Adjust the position of the halo splint to the desired position of the cervical spine.
- Lock all movable parts of the apparatus by tightening all the nuts.
- Sit the patient up. It may be necessary to re-adjust the apparatus before allowing the patient to walk, as some sinking of the plaster jacket may occur when the patient stands up.
  Do not remove the Crutchfield tongs until the final adjustments have been made.

Management of halo traction

1. *Examine the scalp wounds DAILY for the presence of infection.* If a cranial screw site becomes infected, swab the wound to discover the infecting organism and its antibiotic sensitivity, then insert a new sterile screw through an adjacent hole. Tighten the new screw with a torque-limiting screwdriver *before* removing the infected screw.
2. *DAILY for the first week check the tightness of the cranial screws.* Each cranial screw is checked as follows. Hold the cranial screw steady with an ordinary screwdriver while loosening the locking

nut with a spanner. Tighten the cranial screw with a torque-limiting screwdriver preset to 5·5 lb/inches (6·34 kg/cm) until slip occurs. Hold the cranial screw steady, again using an ordinary screwdriver, while re-tightening the locking nut. By holding the cranial screw steady while the locking nut is being loosened and tightened, rotation of the locking nut will not be imparted to the cranial screw.

3. *Wash the patient's hair once or twice each week.*
4. *Check that pressure sores are not developing* under the plaster jacket, especially around the pelvis.
5. *Check that all the locking nuts on the superstructure are tight.*

Halo-pelvic traction

Halo-pelvic traction (Fig. 7.8) consists of a halo splint connected by four vertical extension bars to a steel pelvic hoop. The pelvic hoop in turn is attached to two long threaded steel rods each of which passes through one wing of the ilium (Dewald and Ray, 1970; O'Brien *et al.*, 1971).

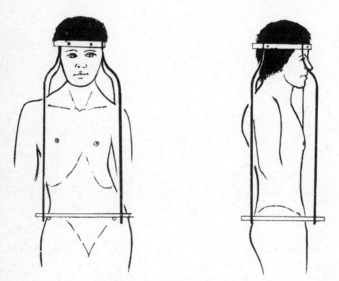

Figure 7.8 Halo-pelvic traction.

This form of skeletal traction may be used to immobilize the spine or to slowly correct or reduce deformities of the spine, such as occur in scoliosis and tuberculosis, before spinal fusion is carried out. The halo-pelvic apparatus remains in place during the operation and for a variable period of time afterwards. Patients in halo-pelvic traction may remain ambulant.

The halo splint is basically similar to that described above under 'halo traction', except that posteriorly the band does not arch upwards to clear the occipital area, and it is drilled and tapped around its perimeter to accept screws for the attachment of the four extension bars.

Each threaded rod transfixes one wing of the ilium, following the ilio-pectineal line beneath the iliacus muscle and passing through four cortices of bone in the thickest portion of the pelvis (Fig. 7.9).

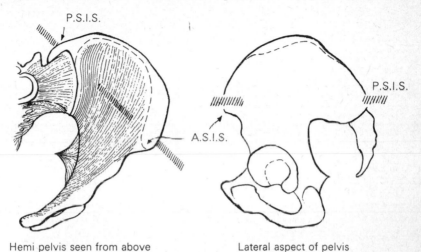

P.S.I.S.

A.S.I.S.

P.S.I.S.

Hemi pelvis seen from above   Lateral aspect of pelvis

Figure 7.9   Halo-pelvic traction. Each threaded rod transfixes one wing of the ilium, passing through four cortices of bone from just above and lateral to the anterior superior iliac spine (A.S.I.S.) to the posterior superior iliac spine (P.S.I.S.) on the same side.

The pelvic hoop, which must be of large enough diameter to allow a gap of 1 to 1½ inches (2·5 to 3·8 cm) between the patient's skin and the hoop, is attached to the threaded rods by four universal clamps. Superiorly the extension bars are attached to the halo splint. Inferiorly they pass through four universal clamps, different from those which clamp the pelvic hoop to the threaded rods, on the pelvic hoop. Locking nuts are placed on each extension bar, one above and the other below the clamp. By adjusting the position of these locking nuts, the effective length of the extension bars can be increased, thus increasing the distance between the halo splint and the pelvic hoop and thereby exerting a distraction force upon the spine.

APPLICATION OF HALO-PELVIC TRACTION
Halo-pelvic traction may be applied under endotracheal anaesthesia or after the administration of Ketamine Hydrochloride (Ketalar, Parke-Davis).*

* See Appendix.

Halo splint, pelvic rods and hoop

Under full aseptic conditions, apply the halo splint as described under 'Halo Traction'.

- Mount a threaded rod in a hand brace.
- Make a small stab wound just above and lateral to the anterior superior iliac spine on each side, in order that the threaded rod will enter bone at the widest part of the ilium.
- Position the drilling jig (Cass and Dwyer, 1969). Place the posterior end of the jig over the posterior superior iliac spine, and then insert the anterior end of the jig through the stab wound *on the same side* until it impinges upon the pelvis just above and lateral to the anterior superior iliac spine. Tighten the jig. The use of the jig ensures the correct positioning of the threaded rods.
- Check the position of the jig by pushing a Steinmann pin through the anterior part of the jig into the ilium.
- Insert the mounted threaded rod into the jig and drill it through the wing of the ilium in an antero-posterior direction, removing the jig when the point of the rod emerges posteriorly from the bony pelvis.
- Insert the second rod through the opposite wing of the ilium in the same manner.
- Apply small dry dressings around the entry and exit wounds.
- Clamp the pelvic hoop to the threaded rods, arranging the hoop to lie evenly around the pelvis in a horizontal plane. The pelvic hoop if possible should lie above the threaded rods as this allows the patient to sit more comfortably without the threaded rods impinging on the thighs. However, to ensure the horizontal positioning of the pelvic hoop, the hoop may lie either above or below the threaded rods on one or both sides.
- Remove the lengths of the threaded rods projecting beyond the pelvic hoop by cutting them with heavy-duty bolt cutters.
- Return the patient to the ward.

Extension bars. Fit the extension bars the following day, after the patient has recovered fully from the anaesthetic. This reduces the incidence of respiratory complications. If the spine is unstable because of the presence of a fracture or fracture-dislocation, apply traction to the halo splint to immobilise the spine until the extension bars are fitted.

- Sit the patient comfortably on a stool.
- Apply traction to the halo splint so that the patient sits erect with his buttocks almost raised from the stool.
- Ensure that the cervical spine is neither flexed nor extended.
- Select four extension bars of adequate length.
- Position the second set of four universal clamps on the pelvic hoop so that they lie at the corners of a square, two antero-laterally and two postero-laterally.
- Check that one locking nut is screwed well up on the lower threaded portion of each extension bar.
- Insert the lower threaded end of each extension bar through one of the universal clamps.
- Select suitable holes on the halo splint at approximately 2, 4, 8 and

10 o'clock, and attach the upper end of each extension bar to the halo splint.

- Carefully adjust the position of the universal clamps on the pelvic hoop so that the extension bars lie evenly disposed on each side of the patient and do not interfere with movement of the upper limbs. The extension bars may have to be contoured, when there is a large rib hump or pelvic obliquity, to avoid pressure on the skin.
- Screw the upper locking nuts down onto the clamps to maintain the correct length of the extension bars before screwing up the lower locking nuts.
- Release the traction on the halo splint.
- If the position of the extension bars is satisfactory, tighten all screws and nuts on the halo splint, extension bars and pelvic hoop with a spanner, Allan key or screwdriver. Remember that the cranial screws on the halo splint must be tightened only with a torque-limiting screwdriver.
- Return the patient to the ward.

Management of halo-pelvic traction

1. *Every patient in halo-pelvic traction must be examined DAILY,* especially while distraction is being carried out, *for the presence of any neurological complications* (see below).
2. *Examine the scalp wounds DAILY for the presence of infection* (see under Halo traction).
3. *DAILY for the first week check the tightness of the cranial screws* (see under Halo traction).
4. *Examine the wounds around the pelvic rods at regular intervals for the presence of infection.* If infection is present, swab the wound to determine the infecting organism and its antibiotic sensitivity. Infection at these sites usually responds rapidly to regular cleansing with an antibacterial solution and systemic antibiotics.
5. Ask the patient if he feels pain around the pelvic rods. Pain may be caused by infection or loosening of the rods.
6. Check that all the screws and nuts on the pelvic hoop and extension bars are tight. This must be carried out twice each week until the apparatus is removed.
7. Wash the patient's hair once or twice each week.
8. *Distraction.* Lengthen the distraction bars each day by loosening the lower locking nuts and then screwing down each of the upper locking nuts by two complete turns. Two complete turns equals 0·1 inch (2·5 mm). Retighten the lower locking nuts.

It has been found that by delaying distraction for one week after the extension bars have been fitted, the incidence of neurological complications is decreased (Manning, 1972).

Distraction is continued until the desired correction has been achieved, the patient suffers painful spasm of the neck muscles, or neurological complications (see below) occur.

Complications of halo-pelvic traction

(See also Complications of skull traction, page 65.)

1. Superficial infection around the pelvic rods and cranial screws.
2. Loosening of the cranial screws and pelvic rods.
3. Psoas spasm which causes difficulty in walking without assistance. It is relieved by removing the pelvic rods (O'Brien *et al.*, 1971).
4. Neurological complications may result from traction lesions of peripheral or cranial nerves or the spinal cord. They may be temporary or permanent.

   Abducent nerve palsy—the patient is unable to move the affected eye in an outward direction. Contraction of the internal rectus muscle eventually leads to internal strabismus and diplopia.

   Glosso-pharyngeal nerve palsy—the patient complains of difficulty in swallowing and may choke. There is loss of sensation to touch and taste over the posterior third of the tongue (Manning, 1972).

   Recurrent laryngeal nerve palsy—hoarseness.

   Hypoglossal nerve palsy—on protrusion, the tongue deviates to the affected side.

   Brachial plexus palsy—either the upper or lower or all of the components of the brachial plexus (C5, C6, C7, C8 and T1) may be involved.

   Spinal cord—paraplegia. This is more likely to occur when congenital scoliosis is being treated.

   When any of the above neurological complications occur, distraction must be discontinued immediately.

   Paraesthesiae in the distribution of the lateral cutaneous nerve of the thigh—may occur following insertion of the pelvic rods. It settles in one to two weeks without any specific measures being taken.
5. Death from respiratory insufficiency.
6. Cervical subluxation C1 on C2. This results from the incorrect application of the appliance with the cervical spine in flexion (Morton and Malins, 1971).
7. Osteoporosis of the vertebrae.

REFERENCES

CASS, C. A. and DWYER, A. F. (1969) A drilling jig for arthrodesis of the hip. *Journal of Bone and Joint Surgery*, **51-B**, 135.

CONE, W. and TURNER, W. G. (1937) The treatment of fracture-dislocation of the cervical vertebrae by skeletal traction and fusion. *Journal of Bone and Joint Surgery*, **19**, 584.

CRUTCHFIELD, W. G. (1933) Skeletal traction for dislocation of the cervical spine. Report of a case. *Southern Surgeon*, **2**, 156.

CRUTCHFIELD, W. G. (1954) Skeletal traction in treatment of injuries to the cervical spine. *Journal of the American Medical Association*, **155**, 29.

DEWALD, R. L. and RAY, R. D. (1970) Skeletal traction for the treatment of severe scoliosis. *Journal of Bone and Joint Surgery*, **52-A**, 233.

MANNING, C. W. S. F. (1972): Personal communication.

MORTON, J. and MALINS, P. (1971) The correction of spinal deformities by halo-pelvic traction. *Physiotherapy*, **57**, 576.

NICKEL, V. L., PERRY, J., GARRETT, A. and HEPPENSTALL, M. (1968) The halo; a spinal skeletal traction fixation device. *Journal of Bone and Joint Surgery*, **50-A**, 1400.

O'BRIEN, J. P., YAU, A. C. M. C., SMITH, T. K. and HODGSON, A. R. (1971) Halo pelvic traction. A preliminary report on a method of external skeletal fixation for correcting deformities and maintaining fixation of the spine. *Journal of Bone and Joint Surgery*, **53-B**, 217.

PERRY, J. and NICKEL, V. L. (1959) Total cervical spine fusion for neck paralysis. *Journal of Bone and Joint Surgery*, **41-A**, 37.

ROGERS, W. A. (1957) Fracture and dislocation of the cervical spine. An end-result study. *Journal of Bone and Joint Surgery*, **39-A**, 341.

THOMPSON, H. (1962) The halo traction apparatus. *Journal of Bone and Joint Surgery*, **44-B**, 655.

WEISL, H. (1971) Unusual complications of skull caliper traction. *Journal of Bone and Joint Surgery*, **54-B**, 143.

8. Spinal supports (thoraco-lumbar and cervical)

Over the years many spinal supports have been designed and later modified. This development has occurred largely in the absence of detailed knowledge of the biomechanics of the spine, with the result that the value, in mechanical terms, of many supports is doubtful. Much work is being done on the biomechanics of the normal spine, but as yet little on the effect of spinal supports on function in either the normal or diseased spine. This work must be increased so that supports which limit the different movements occurring in the different regions of the spine can be designed, manufactured and prescribed with precision. Before spinal supports can be prescribed, knowledge of the functional anatomy of the spine is essential. It must be remembered, however, that the movements which occur in a particular region of the normal spine may differ from those which may be possible in the presence of disease.

FUNCTIONAL ANATOMY OF THE SPINE

Movements occurring in the different regions of the spine

The spinal column is basically a segmented cylindrical structure which subserves three main functions: protection of the spinal cord, support of the trunk, and transmission of the weight of the head, upper limbs and trunk to the pelvis and lower limbs. The segmental nature of the vertebral column confers considerable mobility upon the spine by the summation of the small amounts of movement that can occur between the individual segments.

The movements that occur in the spine are forward flexion, extension, lateral flexion and rotation. The range of movement and the directions in which it can occur differ in each region of the spine, depending upon the anatomical structure of that region.

Cervical spine

In the cervical region the range of forward flexion, extension and lateral flexion is considerable. Rotation mainly occurs between the atlas and axis. Below the level of the axis, the upper articular facets of the posterior articulations face posteriorly and slightly upwards, and the lower facets anteriorly and slightly downwards. This configuration of the articular facets prevents rotation occurring between the individual cervical vertebrae (C2 to C7) without concomitant lateral flexion.

Thoracic spine

In the thoracic region, the ribs limit rotation less than they limit movements in the other directions. The articular facets of the posterior articulations lie in a nearly vertical plane, the upper pair facing posteriorly and very slightly laterally, and the lower pair facing in the opposite direction. This configuration allows up to 6 degrees of rotation between adjacent vertebrae (Gregersen and Lucas, 1967). The centre of axial rotation in the thoracic region lies within or anterior to the intervertebral disc. Lateral flexion in this region is accompanied by some degree of rotation.

Lumbar spine

In the lumbar region, forward flexion, extension and lateral flexion are free, but rotation is limited not so much by the configuration of the articular facets of the posterior articulations which on transverse sections are curved, as by the annulus fibrosus which restricts lateral displacement of adjacent vertebral bodies. The superior articular facets, situated further apart than the lower pair, face medially and slightly posteriorly, while the lower pair face laterally and slightly anteriorly. The centre of axial rotation in the lumbar region lies posterior to the articular processes. Up to 10 degrees of rotation can occur at the thoraco-lumbar junction. A further 10 degrees of rotation can occur between the first and fifth lumbar vertebrae in the sitting position, this being increased to 16 degrees in the standing position (Gregersen and Lucas, 1967). Approximately 6 degrees of rotation, which is always associated with flexion of the fifth lumbar vertebra on the sacrum, can occur at the lumbo-sacral junction (Lumsden and Morris, 1968).

During walking, the pelvis and shoulders rotate in opposite directions, the amount of rotation depending upon the length of each step. Gregersen and Lucas (1967) found that during walking 5 degrees of rotation of the pectoral girdle occurred in one direction measured at the level of the first thoracic vertebra and, at the pelvis, 6 degrees in the opposite direction, the transition point lying between the sixth and eighth thoracic vertebrae. Lumsden and Morris (1968) calculated that approximately 1·5 degrees of rotation occurred at the lumbo-sacral junction during normal walking.

The range of lateral flexion is greater in the upper region of the lumbar spine than in the lower, being maximal at the L3/4 level (Tanz, 1953), whereas the range of forward flexion is greater in the lower region of the lumbar spine than in the upper, being maximal at the L4/5 and L5/S1 levels (Tanz, 1953; Allbrook, 1957). In forward flexion from the standing position, movement occurs both in the lumbar spine and at the hip joints. The distance, therefore, between the finger tips and the floor, on carrying out this manoeuvre varies from one individual to another depending upon the length of the hamstring muscles and the mobility of the lumbar spine. For this reason, the range of lumbar flexion should be tested in both the standing and sitting positions. The lumbar spine is substantially flexed when sitting erect, and the flexion is increased markedly when sitting slumped, the degree of forward flexion between the fourth and fifth lumbar vertebrae actually exceeding that observed during maximal forward bending (Norton and Brown, 1957). As movement of the lumbar spine largely occurs secondary to movements of the lower limbs on the trunk (Troup et al., 1968), absolute immobilisation of the lumbar spine cannot be achieved by external support without severely restricting the movements of the lower limbs.

Vertebral stability and control of spinal movements

The vertebral column depends for its stability upon the structure and integrity of the individual vertebrae and the soft tissues which control and bind them together.

The movement of the vertebral column as a whole is controlled by muscles which bridge many segments, the sacrospinalis muscles, the psoas, the diaphragm, the abdominal muscles and other muscles of the trunk. Movement of individual segments is controlled by muscles which bridge only one or two segments.

The paravertebral muscles can be divided into three groups. The longitudinal group, the sacrospinalis muscles, are most superficial. They bridge many segments and form a large muscular mass which is thickest in the lumbar region. The muscles of the oblique group lie deep to the sacrospinalis muscles and include multifidus which is thickest in the lumbar region, and rotatores which are confined to the thoracic region of the spine. The muscles of the oblique group and the still deeper situated intersegmental group, interspinales and intertransversarii, bridge only one or two segments.

Electromyography of the paravertebral, psoas and abdominal muscles give some indication of their function. The sacrospinalis muscles exhibit some activity when sitting and standing (Morris et al., 1962; Nachemson, 1966), this activity being greater in the lower thoracic and upper lumbar regions of the spine (Joseph and McColl, 1961). They and the oblique group of muscles are also active during forward flexion, this activity being increased if weights are held in the hands (Nachemson, 1966). Activity decreases when the fully flexed spine is at rest, multifidus and rotatores then being inactive. During the early stages of extension of the flexed trunk, there is little electromyographic activity in the paravertebral muscles, extension occurring mainly at the hip joints (Floyd and Silver, 1955). Later this activity increases, but decreases again as the erect position is regained. When extension from the erect position is forced, the sacrospinalis muscles, but not multifidus, are active (Morris *et al.*, 1962).

Lateral flexion from the erect position is accompanied by definite activity in the ipsilateral, but only slight activity in the contralateral, sacrospinalis muscles, suggesting that these muscles assist gravity. Activity is not greatly increased during assumption of the erect position.

In the erect position, the sacrospinalis muscles are generally active during ipsilateral, and the multifidus and rotatores during contralateral rotation (Morris *et al.*, 1962).

Psoas is active when sitting or standing erect, this activity increasing with any deviation of the trunk from the vertical, especially extension and lateral flexion (Keagy *et al.*, 1966; Nachemson, 1966), but decreasing as the erect spine is flexed forward (Nachemson, 1966).

During forward flexion and the early stages of extension of the *flexed* trunk, especially if this action is associated with lifting, considerable forces are generated within the spine, particularly in the lumbo-sacral region. Contraction of the thoracic and abdominal muscles and those of the diaphragm and pelvic floor, raises the pressures within the thoracic and abdominal cavities and converts these cavities into rigid-walled structures, which are capable of transmitting forces produced during bending and lifting, and thereby reducing the forces within the spine (Davis, 1956; Bartelink, 1957). The pressures within the thoracic and abdominal cavities increase as the weight lifted increases (Davis and Troup, 1964). It is calculated that these pressures decrease the force on the lumbo-sacral disc by 30 per cent and on the lower thoracic spine by 50 per cent (Morris *et al.*, 1961). The mechanical advantage of the pressure increases is greatest when the lumbar spine is flexed. These pressure increases thus have their greatest effect during the acceleration phase of lifting before the spine begins to extend (Davis and Troup, 1965).

The rectus abdominis is inactive in standing and sitting (Waters and Morris, 1970). When the trunk is raised from the supine position, the rectus abdominis and the external oblique muscles are active, this activity being greater from 0 to 45 degrees, than from 45 to 90 degrees, the later movement being primarily one of hip flexion. On lowering the trunk, activity is again greater from 45 to 0 degrees (Flint, 1965).

The load on the intervertebral discs in the lumbar region depends upon the position of the trunk and the weight of the body above but largely upon the tension developed by the muscles of the trunk. The pressures within these discs are greatest in the sitting position and are reduced by 30 per cent on standing and by 50 per cent on reclining (Nachemson and Morris, 1964).

THORACO-LUMBAR SPINAL APPLIANCES

Function of spinal appliances

The many different spinal appliances which have been designed can be divided into two groups, supportive and corrective. They are used to relieve pain, to support weakened or paralysed muscles and unstable joints, to immobilise the vertebral column in the best functional position while healing occurs, to prevent the occurrence of deformity, and to correct an existing deformity. The supportive group includes supports made from various fabrics (belts and corsets), rigid spinal braces, and those moulded from leather, plastic, plaster-of-Paris and Plastazote. Those appliances in the corrective group produce an active corrective force in one or more directions. The various functional advantages that have been claimed for these different appliances are difficult to evaluate.

Investigations have been carried out in an attempt to determine the effect of various spinal supports upon the mobility of the spine and the electrical activity of its controlling muscles. However, the results of these investigations may not be applicable to patients suffering from disorders of the spine as the observations were made upon people with normal spines.

Fabric supports restrict only the extremes of forward flexion and extension (Van Leuven and Troup, 1969), and have a variable and unpredictable effect upon rotation at the lumbo-sacral junction (Lumsden and Morris, 1968). They decrease the activity of the paravertebral and abdominal muscles during standing but do not have any significant effect during slow or fast walking (Waters and Morris, 1970). However, when an (inflatable) corset produces sufficient abdominal compression to be uncomfortable, the activity of the abdominal muscles on lifting decreases, indicating that the activity of the thoracic and abdominal muscles can be reduced by external abdominal pressure (Morris et al., 1961).

The presence of an inflated corset also reduces the pressure within the lumbar discs when standing (Nachemson and Morris, 1964). These findings may not be applicable to the fabric supports prescribed for patients.

Long spinal braces, for example the Taylor brace (see below), and the plaster-of-Paris moulded spinal support, increase movement at the lumbo-sacral junction, but decrease movement at the upper levels (Norton and Brown, 1957). Rotation at the lumbo-sacral junction is restricted by short spinal braces when standing, but increased when walking (Lumsden and Morris, 1968). They decrease the activity of the abdominal and paravertebral muscles during standing, but do not have any effect during slow walking. During fast walking the activity of the abdominal muscles is again un-affected, but that of the paravertebral muscles is increased (Waters and Morris, 1970).

In spite of the apparent mechanical deficiencies of spinal sup-ports many patients obtain symptomatic relief from their use. This relief may be psychological, or may result from abdominal com-pression, from support of a pendulous abdomen and a concomitant decrease in lumbar lordosis, from a change in the amount of movement occurring in different regions of the spine, from a decrease in activity of the various associated muscle groups, from local support of the sacro-iliac joints and ilio-lumbar ligaments, or from a combination of all these factors. It is interesting that sub-jective support can be obtained by the application of non-elastic adhesive strapping to the lumbar and gluteal regions of the back.

SUPPORTIVE SPINAL APPLIANCES

Fabric spinal supports (Spinal belts and corsets)

Spinal belts and corsets are the most commonly prescribed spinal supports (Perry, 1970). The majority of these supports are made from jean (twilled weave Egyptian cotton), coutil (herring-bone weave Egyptian cotton) or canvas (plain weave American cotton). They can be made also from duck (light canvas), rayon, nylon or airtex (open weave cotton). They are reinforced as necessary with bone or metal strips. Corsets extend further down over the buttocks and upper thighs than do belts to give a smoother contour, and therefore are prescribed for women. Belts are prescribed for men.

These supports encircle the sacral region and extend a variable distance upwards, the term applied to them (sacro-iliac, lumbo-sacral, thoraco-lumbar) depending upon their depth posteriorly (see below). In front they are fastened with straps and buckles, eyelets and laces or hooks and eyes. In addition a fulcrum strap (Figs. 8.1 and 8.2), broad posteriorly where it is attached to the mid-line, and narrowing towards the front, fastens in the front with a buckle. Elastic insets may be let into the upper and lower margins to ease the fitting over the costal margin and around the buttocks re-spectively.

Fabric supports, even when reinforced with metal strips, do not immobilise the spine; they only restrict the extremes of forward and lateral flexion, and extension. They probably function by supplying subjective support and by reminding the patient to avoid movements which may bring on or exacerbate his symptoms.

A sacro-iliac support is 2 to 6 inches (5 to 15 cm) deep pos-teriorly and basically consists of a wide belt of leather or fabric which encircles the pelvis, passing between the greater trochanters and the iliac crests on each side. It is fastened anteriorly by straps and buckles or hooks. Perineal straps may be added to prevent the support from riding upwards.

A lumbo-sacral support (Figs. 8.1 and 8.2) is 8 to 16 inches (20 to 40 cm) deep posteriorly. It extends up to the thoraco-lumbar junction posteriorly and covers the entire abdomen anteriorly. It has a closely fitting fulcrum strap, attached posteriorly, which passes around the pelvis between the greater trochanters and the iliac crests and buckles firmly in the region of the symphysis pubis, thus obtaining a grip on the pelvis and giving a stable foundation to the support. Flexible or rigid vertical metal strips are incorporated posteriorly on each side of the spinous processes to reinforce the support and to provide a wide stable area posteriorly from which the support can act on the abdomen. Further vertical metal strips can be added to increase rigidity. To ease pressure on the costal

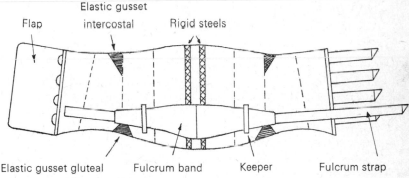

Figure 8.1 Lumbo-sacral support. Typical minimum depth at the centre back is that from the thoraco-lumbar junction to the middle of the sacrum.

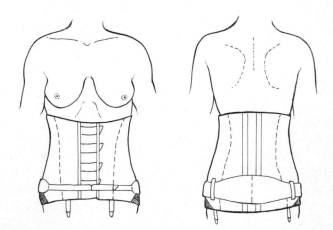

Figure 8.2 Lumbo-sacral support can be fitted with suspenders or groin straps.

margin, elastic gussets can be let into the upper edge. Perineal straps or suspenders may be fitted to prevent the support from riding upwards. The support is adjusted by straps and buckles or eyelets and laces. A 'quick release' panel of hooks and eyes is often incorporated.

A thoraco-lumbar support is more than 16 inches (40 cm) deep posteriorly, and extends upwards over the scapulae. Padded shoulder straps which must be kept fairly tight are fitted. Otherwise the basic construction is identical with that of the lumbo-sacral support. It provides considerable support.

When a support is worn by an obese, heavy-breasted woman, a ridge of skin and subcutaneous fat can be trapped between the upper edge of the support and the lower edge of her brassière. This difficulty can be overcome by the addition of brassière cups to the support, or by advising the woman to wear a 'long-line' brassière.

FITTING OF FABRIC SPINAL SUPPORTS
Check the support
- The support must be adequate for its intended function.
- It must extend well down to the symphysis pubis.
- It must fit firmly and smoothly over the greater trochanters, iliac crests and buttocks.
- The posterior steel strips must follow closely the curves of the sacrum and spine.
- It must not interfere with hip flexion and sitting.
- It must not ride upwards.
- It must be comfortable. Some patients who have not worn a support before may find it uncomfortable at first. They should be advised to gradually lengthen the time they wear it, as they would do with new shoes.

Instruct the patient
The fulcrum strap must always be firmly buckled.
The other abdominal straps or laces must be tightened firmly also, although to ease pressure over the costal margin and thighs the upper and lowermost fastenings may be left slightly loose.

Immediate lumbar supports

A fabric support made to fit an individual patient takes time to manufacture. An easily made and cheap 'instant' lumbar support has been described by Nichols *et al.* (1966). A length of Tubigrip body bandage of either single or double thickness, extending from the nipples to the upper thighs, is rolled onto the patient. With the patient lying prone, sitting or standing, whichever is the most comfortable, 6 to 12 thicknesses of 6 to 8 inches (15 to 20 cm) wide plaster-of-Paris bandage are applied over the spine from the thoraco-lumbar junction to the sacrum. The top and bottom of the Tubigrip bandage are turned back and fixed down.

Rigid spinal braces

All spinal braces, except the anterior hyperextension brace described later, are constructed on the basis of a metal frame which takes firm support from the pelvis. Metal uprights, joined together by various cross bars, are attached to the pelvic support. Devices to apply pressure over the abdomen and over the front of the shoulders are provided. The metal frame is padded with felt and covered with leather.

The metal frame must have a firm foundation on the pelvis to hold the appliance in contact with the body, and to distribute the body weight, transmitted by the uprights, over a large area. This can be obtained by using a pelvic band or a moulded pelvic corset. A pelvic band is made from flat metal bars which encircle the posterior and lateral aspects of the pelvis and press upon the sacrum. These metal bars extend for a variable distance towards the midline anteriorly in different types of braces. A moulded pelvic corset (Fig. 8.8) gives a firm grip around the pelvis. The corset may be made of leather or plastic. A negative cast of the pelvis and abdomen is taken with plaster of Paris or Plastazote, from which a positive plaster model is made. The leather or plastic is moulded over the plaster model.

The metal uprights attached to the pelvic support extend upwards for varying distances depending upon the length of spine to be supported. There are two uprights posteriorly lying on each side of the spinous processes—the back lever. To obtain more rigidity, further uprights can be attached laterally or anteriorly. The uprights are joined together by horizontal cross bars. When lateral or anterior uprights are present, the cross bar in the thoracic region extends anteriorly around the trunk below the axillae (Fig. 8.4).

Abdominal support is obtained by an abdominal plate (Figs. 8.3 and 8.5) attached by straps and buckles to the metal frame, or by a fabric corset (Fig. 8.4). Pressure over the front of the shoulders to hold them back into the brace can be obtained by using padded shoulder straps or clavicular pads which curve upwards and press on the chest wall in the infra-clavicular region.

There are many spinal braces with the same basic construction but called by different names. Some braces have withstood the test of time, while the existence of others is perpetuated by the written word (Perry, 1970). Described below are some of the more commonly used spinal braces. The descriptions used are those found in the Surgical Appliances Contract 1972 of the Department of Health and Social Security.

Taylor spinal brace (Fig. 8.3)

In 1863, C. F. Taylor described a spinal brace, for use in the treatment of tuberculosis of the spine, which can be considered as

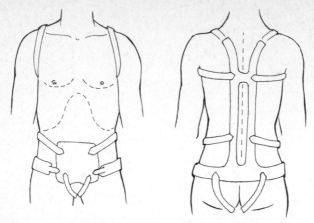

Figure 8.3   Taylor spinal brace.

the prototype of all spinal braces designed to support the thoraco-lumbar spine. It consists of a wide straight spring-steel pelvic band which extends forward in front of the anterior superior iliac spines. The pelvic band is completed anteriorly with leather straps and buckles. There are two parallel posterior uprights connected at the level of the scapulae by a cross bar made from a thin plate of moulded steel. Above this level the uprights gently angle outwards towards the shoulders. The steel frame is padded with a thin layer of felt and covered with leather.

Shoulder straps, covered by upward extensions of the leather covering the posterior uprights, pass from the uprights over the shoulders and back under the axillae to be attached to the cross bar. Abdominal support is provided by a rigid, padded, leather abdominal plate, extending between the umbilicus and the symphysis pubis, which is attached below to the pelvic band and above to the posterior uprights by two straps which pass backwards around the loins. Groin straps are fitted also.

The Taylor brace limits forward flexion, extension and lateral flexion of the thoraco-lumbar region of the spine and, to some extent, rotation of the lumbar and lower thoracic regions of the spine. It increases movement at the lumbo-sacral junction (Norton and Brown, 1957).

Fisher spinal brace (Fig. 8.4)
The Fisher spinal brace was described originally in 1886. It consists of a metal pelvic band to which two metal pelvic hoops, one on each side, are attached. These pelvic hoops arch over the iliac crests. There are two posterior uprights and two adjustable lateral uprights. A transverse metal bar, at the level of the inferior angles of the scapulae, joins the posterior and lateral uprights and ends anteriorly in axillary crutches. All the metal parts except the lateral uprights are padded with a thin layer of felt and covered with leather.

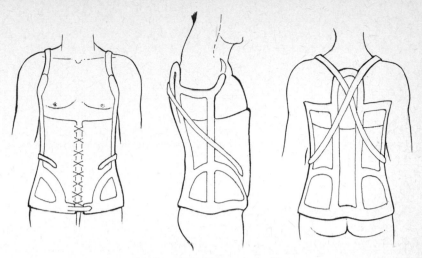

Figure 8.4 Fisher spinal brace.

Abdominal support is provided by a fabric corset which extends forward from the lateral uprights and fastens in the mid-line anteriorly. Well padded shoulder straps pass up from the tips of the axillary crutches, over the shoulders, cross posteriorly, and then swing forwards again to buckle on the front of the corset on each side level with the iliac crests.

The axillary crutches are not designed to bear weight. If they press into the axillae, nerve palsies will result.

The Fisher spinal brace limits forward flexion and extension of the lower thoracic and upper lumbar regions of the spine. Lateral flexion is limited more than with the Taylor spinal brace. Rotation of the thoracic spine is limited also.

Thomas or Jones spinal brace (Fig. 8.5)

This type of spinal brace was designed originally by H. O. Thomas.

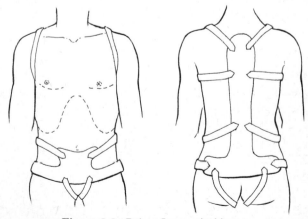

Figure 8.5 Robert Jones spinal brace.

It was used extensively by Sir Robert Jones instead of a plaster-of-Paris moulded support, for the ambulant treatment of spinal tuberculosis (Jones and Lovett, 1923).

It consists of a large padded pelvic strap which is attached posteriorly to a padded, leather-covered metal frame. Abdominal support is provided by an abdominal pad to which are buckled waist, pelvic and groin straps. Shoulder straps pass from the metal frame over the shoulders and under the axillae to be reattached to the metal frame at the level of the inferior angles of the scapulae.

FITTING OF LONG SPINAL BRACES

- Tighten the pelvic band and ensure that the pelvic band or pelvic corset fits snugly around the pelvis.
- Check that the posterior metal uprights follow closely the contour of the spine.
- After checking the posterior uprights, tighten the shoulder straps if fitted.
- Fasten the groin and waist straps, abdominal plate or fabric corset if fitted.
- Check that the axillary crutches, if fitted, do not press into the axillae.
- (With a Jones spinal brace, when the patient stands with a good posture, it should be possible to slip two fingers between the back lever and the upper part of the spine.)

Anterior hyperextension spinal brace (Fig. 8.6)
This type of brace utilises a completely different method of construction from the above spinal braces. It was described originally by Hoadley in 1896, who used it to provide mechanical support 'of the spinal column between the middle of the lumbar and the middle of the thoracic regions'. It employs the principle of three-point action of a bending force. Numerous modifications to this brace have been made, but that of Baker (1942) is described here.

The anterior hyperextension spinal brace consists basically of a rectangular metal frame, the short sides of which fit over the front

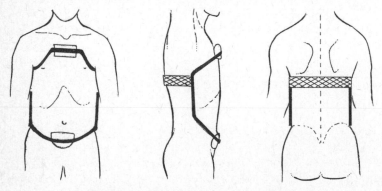

Figure 8.6   Anterior hyperextension brace.

of the thorax and abdomen, in the pectoral and inguinal regions respectively, while the longer sides lie in the mid-axillary line. Pads, hinged on the metal frame, lie over the pubis and upper sternum. An elastic strap passes posteriorly from the side arms over the thoracic spine and is kept sufficiently tight to hold the brace against the patient's body. Additional pelvic and thoracic straps may be added to keep the brace in position.

Moulded spinal supports

Moulded spinal supports fit the contours of the trunk and distribute the body weight over a very large area. They can be made from leather, plastic, plaster-of-Paris or Plastazote. Their rigidity will depend upon the material used in their construction. A leather support can be reinforced by attaching metal bands. A Plastazote support is less rigid than a plaster-of-Paris or plastic support, but it is light and comfortable to wear, and can be moulded directly onto the patient (see Chapter 16), as can plaster-of-Paris. Leather and plastic supports require to be moulded over a positive model of the patient and therefore are more expensive and take longer to make than do those made from plaster-of-Paris or Plastazote.

These supports must extend from the symphysis pubis to the upper sternum anteriorly and be accurately fitted around the pelvis. They are cut low posteriorly (Fig. 8.7).

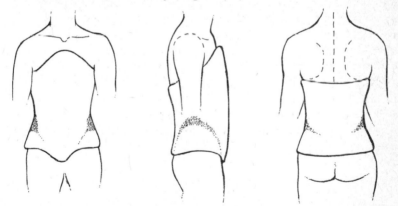

Figure 8.7 Moulded spinal jacket, extends from the upper sternum to the symphysis pubis anteriorly and is cut lower posteriorly.

PRESCRIBING A SUPPORTIVE SPINAL APPLIANCE

It is impossible here to give detailed indications for the prescription of the various spinal supports, as they depend upon the underlying spinal disability and its site and extent, the intensity of the patient's symptoms and their response to other forms of treatment, the patient's age and sex, whether the appliance is to be worn permanently or only for a limited time, and the function required of the appliance (Berger, 1969).

Before a spinal support is prescribed, it is imperative that an accurate history is taken, a detailed physical and radiological examination is performed, and other special investigations are carried out in an attempt to diagnose accurately the cause and site of the patient's symptoms. Treatment in all cases must be directed towards the underlying cause of the symptoms which often may be relieved by means other than a spinal support. When symptoms persist or change, in spite of apparent adequate treatment, the patient must be reassessed carefully, as the symptoms may be due to a pathological condition, for example tuberculosis or neoplasia, which could not be detected initially.

Spinal appliances are prescribed commonly under a proper name, which name may be that of the original designer or someone who has modified the appliance. In addition many appliances, although called by the same proper name, may differ considerably in construction from place to place, and appliances of the same design and construction may be called by different names in different places. It is important therefore to describe accurately the appliance required, the movements which the appliance is intended to control, and to ensure that the appliance supplied to the patient fits correctly and fulfils its intended function.

Fabric spinal supports

Sacro-iliac support. This support may be prescribed for the rare cases of sacro-iliac strain.

Lumbo-sacral support. These supports are prescribed commonly in the management of chronic low back pain which may be due to a variety of causes, such as generalised degenerative changes affecting the intervertebral discs and posterior articulations, prolapsed intervertebral disc in the later stages after the acute symptoms have subsided, spondylolysis, spondylolisthesis, spinal instability, osteoporosis, minor compression fractures, and following some spinal operations such as spinal fusion.

Thoraco-lumbar support. These are prescribed instead of rigid spinal braces when the patient's symptoms arise from the thoracic or upper lumbar regions of the spine, from conditions such as generalised degenerative changes, senile kyphosis, osteoporosis, minor compression fractures, and spinal infections in the elderly.

Rigid spinal braces

Rigid spinal braces are more effective in reducing movement in the lower thoracic and upper lumbar regions of the spine than fabric supports. It must be remembered, however, that movement in the adjacent regions of the spine, especially the lumbo-sacral junction, tends to be increased (Norton and Brown, 1957), and this increase in movement may give rise to pain, particularly if degenerative changes are present.

Fisher, Taylor and Jones spinal braces. All these spinal braces limit, to some degree, forward flexion, extension, lateral flexion and rotation in the thoraco-lumbar region of the spine, the Fisher spinal brace being the most effective, and the Jones the least. These spinal braces are used in the ambulant management of tuberculosis of the lower thoracic and upper lumbar regions of the spine, the more severe vertebral compression fractures, vertebral osteochondritis and osteoporosis, and marked weakness of the trunk musculature.

Anterior hyperextension spinal brace. This brace is uncomfortable if the pressure exerted over the thoracic spine is too great. It was designed to provide extension, but is more comfortable when used merely to prevent excessive forward flexion. Conditions which can be treated with this brace are compression fractures of the vertebral bodies and ankylosing spondylitis.

Moulded spinal supports

Moulded leather or plastic spinal supports are reserved usually for the management of severe deformities of the spine from any cause for which it would be impossible to manufacture and fit a fabric support or a rigid spinal brace.

Moulded spinal supports of plaster-of-Paris or Plastazote are used when the need for a support is temporary.

CORRECTIVE SPINAL APPLIANCES

Milwaukee spinal brace (Fig. 8.8)
The Milwaukee spinal brace (Blount *et al.*, 1958) is an active corrective spinal brace used almost exclusively in the ambulant treatment of structural scoliosis, the aim being to postpone, temporarily or permanently, the need for operation. It is used also in the post-operative period. This brace is used occasionally in the management of ankylosing spondylitis and tuberculosis of the upper thoracic region of the spine. In these later two instances, a pressure pad (see below) is not necessary.

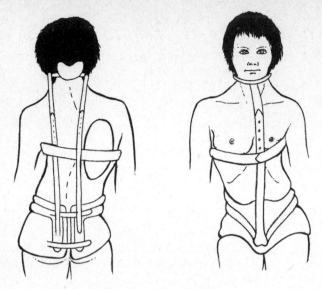

Figure 8.8   Milwaukee brace.

It consists of a moulded leather or Ortholene pelvic corset which fits snugly over the iliac crests, around the waist, and curves upward in front to support the abdomen. It is cut lower at the sides to avoid pressure on the costal margin. Metal side bars are attached to the leather pelvic corset to form a base from which one anterior and two posterior metal uprights pass upwards to a padded ring around the neck. These uprights are adjustable to allow for growth. Anterior and posterior bars with padded submental and occipital pieces are attached to the ring around the neck.

Rib rotation is corrected by a pressure pad located over the rib prominences. The pressure pad is fixed to a single, heavy, broad leather strap which is attached to the uprights at the desired level by stud fastenings. The leather strap is passed over the posterior bar on the convex side so that the pressure is applied directly from the lateral side. To avoid pressure on a breast, the leather strap can be attached to an outrigger on the anterior bar.

Because of the close moulding of the pelvic corset, the brace has to be remade as growth occurs.

FITTING OF A MILWAUKEE SPINAL BRACE

The correct prescribing, manufacture and fitting of a Milwaukee spinal brace is highly specialised, and should be carried out only by experienced surgeons and appliance makers (Orthotists). Outlined below are some important points about the correct fitting of a Milwaukee spinal brace.

- The pelvic corset must fit snugly about the waist above the iliac crests.
- It must be possible at all times to pass a finger between the chin and the submental piece.

- When the patient stands erect and the pressure pads are fitted, he must be able to raise his chin and occiput from the head support at the same time.
- With the head resting upon its supports, the patient must be able to move the chest away from the lateral pressure pad.

If the brace is fitted as outlined above, pressure sores over the chin and occiput, hypoplasia of the mandible and adverse effects upon the incisor teeth will be avoided. Meralgia paraesthetica can occur during the wearing of a Milwaukee spinal brace (Moe and Kettleson, 1970).

CERVICAL SPINAL APPLIANCES

The head is balanced upon the cervical spine by the action of the neck muscles. The cervical spine exhibits a considerable range of movement in all directions. Inflammatory conditions or mechanical derangements of the cervical spine are associated commonly with spasm of the neck muscles and pain. This spasm and pain may be relieved by heat, massage and exercises, but occasionally immobiliz-ation of the cervical spine combined with support of the head to relieve pressure upon the cervical vertebrae, intervertebral discs and joints, and the cervical nerves is required. This can be achieved by spinal traction (see Chapter 7) or by external splintage of the neck.

To immobilize and relieve pressure upon the cervical spine, an external support must be shaped to fit the contours of the lower jaw and occiput, the shoulders, clavicles and sternum and the upper thoracic spine. In the presence of a lesion of the uppermost part of the cervical spine, the forehead also must be included in the support. The inclusion of the thoracic spine and trunk depends upon the level, extent and severity of the lesion of the cervical spine.

For adequate immobilization of a lesion above the level of the sixth thoracic vertebrae, the cervical spine must be immobilized. This is achieved by attaching a cervical support to a long spinal brace, or by prescribing a Milwaukee spinal brace.

Felt or foam rubber collar

This type of collar consists of a length of orthopaedic felt or foam rubber covered with stockinette. It is useful in an emergency or when a temporary support is required, for example following muscle strain. It is prepared as follows:

- Cut a strip of orthopaedic felt or foam rubber measuring 18 inches by 8 inches (45·75 cm by 20·0 cm) and fold it in half lengthways.
- Cover the felt or foam rubber with stockinette, leaving the ends long, to act as ties.

Thomas's collar

Many different cervical supports are called 'Thomas's Collars'. The original cervical support described by Hugh Owen Thomas was made from sheet metal covered with felt and sheepskin. The sheet metal, the edges of which were flared out, reached from the chin to the sternum anteriorly, from the base of the neck to the occiput posteriorly, and was long enough to encircle the neck. The support was fastened securely around the neck, rested upon the chest and shoulders and supported the chin, jaw and occiput.

Thick plastic sheet is used commonly today instead of metal. These collars (Fig. 8.9) are 'ready-made' and are supplied in different

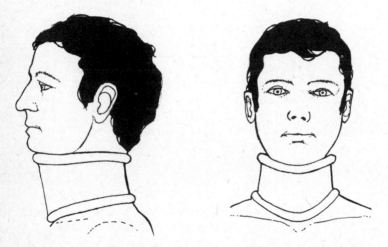

Figure 8.9   Thomas cervical collar.

sizes or are adjustable. Great care must be taken to ensure that they are fastened securely around the neck, rest upon the chest and shoulders and support the chin, jaw and occiput. Often they are fitted incorrectly and do not support the cervical spine at all.

Moulded cervical supports

1. *Plastazote*

Plastazote, a foamed polyethylene, is easily moulded after being heated at 140° C. for 5 minutes in a hot-air oven. After heating it is moulded around the patient's neck, and in this way accurately fitting cervical supports, holding the patient's head in the most comfortable position, can be made rapidly (see Chapter 16).

2. *Polythene*

Supports made from polythene (Fig. 8.10) are used usually for immobilization of the cervical spine after operation. However, unlike Plastazote, a plaster model over which the polythene is moulded, must be made first.

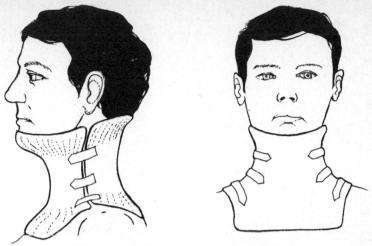

Figure 8.10   Moulded polythene cervical collar.

Cervical braces

There are many different types of cervical brace; one such is illustrated in Figure 8.11. It consists of padded chin and occiput supports attached by adjustable uprights to padded chest and back plates. It is easy to apply and adjust. It can be applied prior to radiological examination when bony injury to the cervical spine is suspected.

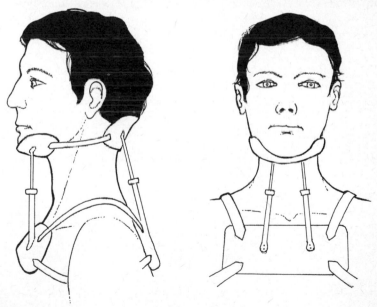

Figure 8.11   Cervical brace. This consists of a lined chin cup and occipital plate attached by four adjustable turnbuckles to two lined plastic plates, one anteriorly and one posteriorly. There are in addition two axillary and shoulder straps, and two straps connecting the chin cup and occipital plate.

Minerva jacket

In the presence of a lesion of the uppermost part of the cervical spine, the forehead also must be included in any external support. The Minerva jacket made from plaster-of-Paris (Fig. 8.12) is used commonly in such situations. The halo traction arrangement (see Chapter 7) may be used also.

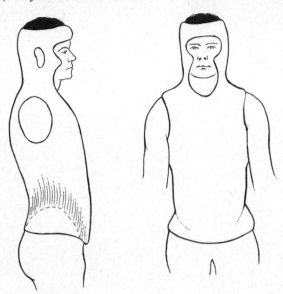

Figure 8.12   Minerva plaster-of-Paris jacket.

REFERENCES

ALLBROOK, D. (1957) Movements of the lumbar spinal column. *Journal of Bone and Joint Surgery*, **39-B**, 339.

BAKER, L. D. (1942) Rhizomelic spondylosis. *Journal of Bone and Joint Surgery*, **24**, 827.

BARTELINK, D. L. (1957) The role of abdominal pressure in relieving the pressure on the lumbar intervertebral discs. *Journal of Bone and Joint Surgery*, **39-B**, 718.

BERGER, N. (1969) Terminology in Spinal Orthotics, p. 44. Spinal Orthotics: A Report Sponsored by the Committee on Prosthetic Research and Development of the Division of Engineering, National Research Council, National Academy of Sciences, Washington, D.C., Chairman, H. Elftman.

BLOUNT, W. P., SCHMIDT, A. C. and Bidwell, R. G. (1958) Making the Milwaukee brace. *Journal of Bone and Joint Surgery*, **40-A**, 526.

DAVIS, P. R. (1956) Variations of the human intra-abdominal pressures during weight-lifting in different postures. *Journal of Anatomy*, **90**, 601.

DAVIS, P. R. and TROUP, J. D. G. (1964) Pressures in the trunk cavities when pulling, pushing and lifting. *Ergonomics*, **7**, 465.

DAVIS, P. R. and TROUP, J. D. G. (1965) Effects on the trunk of handling heavy loads in different postures p. 323. Proceedings of 2nd International Ergonomics Association Congress. Dortmund 1964.

FISHER, F. R. (1886) Orthopaedic surgery; the treatment of deformities. In *International Encyclopaedia of Surgery*, edited by Ashurst, J., Jnr. Vol. 6, p. 1080, Fig. 1509 and p. 1082, Fig. 1510. New York. W. Wood.

FLINT, M. M. (1965) Abdominal muscle involvement during the performance of various forms of sit-up exercises. *American Journal of Physical Medicine*, **44**, 224.

FLOYD, W. F. and SILVER, P. H. S. (1955) The functions of the erectores spinae muscles in certain movements and postures in man. *Journal of Physiology*, **129**, 184.

GREGERSEN, G. G. and LUCAS, D. B. (1967) An in vivo study of the axial rotation of the human thoraco-lumbar spine. *Journal of Bone and Joint Surgery*, **49-A**, 247.

HOADLEY, A. E. (1896) Spine-brace. *Transactions of the American Orthopaedic Association*, **8**, 164.

JONES, R. and LOVETT, R. W. (1923) *Orthopaedic Surgery*, p. 236. London: Henry Frowde and Hodder & Stoughton.

JOSEPH, J. and McCOLL, I. (1961) Electromyography of muscles of posture: posterior vertebral muscles in males. *Journal of Physiology*, **157**, 33.

KEAGY, R. D., BRUMLICK, J. and BERGAN, J. J. (1966) Direct electromyography of the psoas major muscle in man. *Journal of Bone and Joint Surgery*, **48-A**, 1377.

LUMSDEN, R. M. and MORRIS, J. M. (1968) An in vivo study of axial rotation and immobilisation at the lumbo-sacral joint. *Journal of Bone and Joint Surgery*, **50-A**, 1591.

MOE, J. H. and KETTLESON, D. N. (1970) Idiopathic scoliosis. *Journal of Bone and Joint Surgery*, **52-A**, 1509.

MORRIS, J. M., LUCAS, D. B. and BRESLER, B. (1961) Role of the trunk in stability of the spine. *Journal of Bone and Joint Surgery*, **43-A**, 327.

MORRIS, J. M., BENNER, G. and LUCAS, D. B. (1962) An electromyographic study of the intrinsic muscles of the back in man. *Journal of Anatomy*, **96**, 509.

NACHEMSON, A. (1966) Electromyographic studies on the vertebral portion of the psoas muscle. *Acta Orthopaedica Scandinavica*, **37**, 177.

NACHEMSON, A. and MORRIS, J. M. (1964) In vivo measurements of intra-discal pressure: discometry, a method for the determination of pressure in the lower lumbar discs. *Journal of Bone and Joint Surgery*, **46-A**, 1077.

NICHOLS, P. J. R., McCAY, G. and BRADFORD, A. (1966) Immediate lumbar supports. *British Medical Journal*, **ii**, 707.

NORTON, P. L. and BROWN, T. (1957) Immobilising efficiency of back braces: their effect on the posture and motion of the lumbo-sacral spine. *Journal of Bone and Joint Surgery*, **39-A**, 111.

PERRY, J. (1970) The use of external support in the treatment of low-back pain. *Journal of Bone and Joint Surgery*, **52-A**, 1440.

SURGICAL APPLIANCES CONTRACT 1972 (MHM 50), Department of Health and Social Services (D.S.B.4A), Government Buildings, Block I, Warbreck Hill Road, Blackpool.

TANZ, S. S. (1953) Motion of the lumbar spine: a roentgenologic study. *American Journal of Roentgenology*, **69**, 399.

TAYLOR, C. F. (1863) On the mechanical treatment of Pott's disease of the spine. *Transactions of the New York State Medical Society*, **6**, 67.

TROUP, J. D. G., HOOD, C. A. and CHAPMAN, A. E. (1968) Measurements of the sagittal mobility of the lumbar spine and hips. *Annals of Physical Medicine*, **9**, 308.

VAN LEUVEN, R. M. and TROUP, J. D. G. (1969) The 'instant' lumbar corset. *Physiotherapy*, **55**, 499.

WATERS, R. L. and MORRIS, J. M. (1970) Effect of spinal supports on the electrical activity of muscles of the trunk. *Journal of Bone and Joint Surgery*, **52-A**, 51.

9. Splinting for congenital dislocation of the hip

The detection of the unstable hip as soon as possible after birth, and its prompt treatment, are vital. There is no direct evidence that every unstable hip at birth will, if untreated, become a dislocated hip, but if every hip that is found to be unstable at birth is treated, established dislocation of the hip virtually disappears (Rosen, 1962).

Unstable hips at birth are diagnosed clinically. All doctors who work with the new-born must know how to detect an unstable hip. Barlow (1962) found only 159 unstable hips in 9000 births, an incidence of 18 per 1000 (as opposed to 1·5 per 1000 for the incidence of established dislocation of the hip in Western Europe). This means that many normal hips will be examined before an unstable hip is found.

CLINICAL TESTS FOR UNSTABLE HIPS

Barlow's test (1962)

This test must be carried out within two to three days of birth, in a warm room and preferably after the child has been fed, when he will be relaxed and contented. The examiner's hands must be warm. The test is carried out in two stages.

> STAGE ONE
> ● Remove the child's nappy.
> ● Place the child supine on a warm firm surface with its legs pointing towards you.
> ● Hold the knees fully flexed, with the flexed legs in the palms of your hands, and with the middle finger of each hand on the greater trochanter and the thumb on the inner aspect of the thigh opposite the lesser trochanter (Fig. 9.1).
> ● Flex the hips to a right angle and abduct them to 45 degrees.
> ● Press forwards *in turn* with the middle finger of each hand on the greater trochanter and attempt to lift the femoral head into the acetabulum.

The test is positive when the joint is dislocated and the femoral head returns to the acetabulum with a palpable and often audible clunk or jerk. The clunk or jerk is due to the femoral head snapping

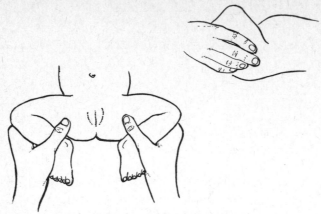

Figure 9.1   Barlow's test.

back over the posterior rim of the acetabulum into the socket. This must not be confused with ligamentous clicking, which can often be elicited from a baby's normal hip.

STAGE TWO
- Continue to hold the lower limbs as described above.
- Press backwards *in turn* with each thumb on the inner side of the thigh. If the femoral head slips backwards onto the posterior lip of the acetabulum or actually dislocates, the hip is unstable.
- In doubtful cases, firmly hold the pelvis with one hand, with the thumb on the pubis and the fingers under the sacrum, while performing the above test on one hip with the opposite hand.
- Examine the second hip in the same way.

This test is reliable and can be used up to the age of six months, by which time the femora have become so long that it is difficult to reach the greater trochanters with the tips of the middle fingers.

Ortolani's test

This test was described by Ortolani in 1948 for use in children between three and nine months old. It is not entirely satisfactory in the new-born (Barlow, 1962).

PROCEDURE:
- Lay the child supine on a warm firm surface with its legs pointing towards you.
- Flex the hips and knees to a right angle with the knees touching and the hips in slight internal rotation.
- Hold one leg steady. With the other knee in the palm of your hand (with

the thumb over the inner side of the knee, and with the other fingers over the greater trochanter), exert gentle pressure in a latero-medial direction with the fingers and at the same time slowly abduct the hip through 90 degrees, until the outer side of the knee touches the couch. When the test is positive, somewhere in the 90 degree arc of abduction reduction of the dislocation will occur and the head of the femur will slip into the acetabulum with a visible and palpable movement—a clunk or jerk.

The tests described above are generally reliable, but they may be misleading in certain situations. When limited abduction of a hip is present due to contraction of its adductor muscles, a clunk may not be elicited. However the presence of limitation of abduction itself may indicate dislocation of that hip. 'Clinks' as opposed to clunks or jerks can often be elicited on manipulation of the normal hips of the new-born.

The incidence of unstable hips decreases in the first few weeks after birth. Nelson (1966) found, on the examination of 866 live births, an incidence of 15·9 per cent soon after birth which fell to 7 per cent seven to ten days after birth, and to 0·35 per cent at three weeks. The decrease in the incidence of unstable hips in the weeks immediately after birth gives rise to some controversy as to whether an unstable hip at birth should be treated immediately or whether only those which are still unstable some weeks after birth should be treated. It is not within the scope of this book to discuss the indications for treatment. Generally, however, it is better to err on the side of over-treatment, as long as the treatment is carried out correctly, and as long as the treatment does not give rise to any complications.

X-RAY EXAMINATION

Ossification in the capital epiphysis of the femur is not present at birth and therefore the capital epiphysis cannot be demonstrated radiologically. This makes the radiological identification of a dislocated hip in the young child difficult. However, the ossific nucleus of the femoral head can be seen radiologically in 78 per cent of normal hips at six months of age and in 99 per cent at one year (Wynne-Davies, 1970).

Under six months of age

Andrén and von Rosen (1958) described a technique for use in this age group in which an antero-posterior X-ray is taken with the child supine and with both lower limbs in full medial rotation and 45 degrees of abduction.

When the head of the femur is dislocated, the upward prolongation of the long axis of the shaft of the femur points towards
the anterior superior iliac spine and crosses the midline in the lower
lumbar region of the spine (Fig. 9.2). When the hip is not dislocated,

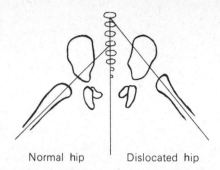

Normal hip   Dislocated hip

Figure 9.2   Antero-posterior X-ray with lower limbs in full medial rotation and
45° abduction in child under six months.

the upward prolongation of the long axis of the shaft of the femur
points towards the lateral margin of the acetabulum and crosses the
posterior part of the pelvis in the region of the sacro-iliac joint
(Fig. 9.2).

As a dislocated hip may reduce with abduction, it is possible to
obtain a false negative result with this technique.

Over six months of age

Once the ossific nucleus of the femoral head is present, standard
antero-posterior X-rays of the pelvis and hips, with the legs together
and in neutral rotation, can be used.

In a normal hip, the ossific nucleus of the femoral head lies below
the horizontal line (of Hilgenreiner) passing through the tri-radiate
cartilages of the acetabula, and medial to the vertical line (of Perkins)
passing through the outer lip of the acetabulum, perpendicular to the
above horizontal line (Fig. 9.3).

When the head of the femur is dislocated, the ossific nucleus of
the head tends to lie lateral to the vertical line and above the
horizontal line (Fig. 9.3).

**Further radiological findings in congenital dislocation
of the hip** (Fig. 9.3)

The ossific nucleus of the dislocated hip is smaller, or its appearance
is delayed, compared with the normal side.

The angle between the horizontal line of Hilgenreiner and the line
of the acetabular roof (acetabular angle or index) is greater than
35 degrees.

Shenton's line is broken.

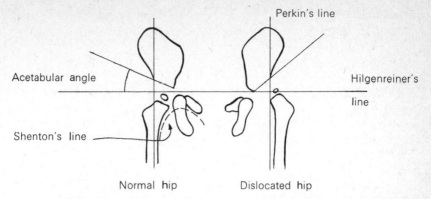

Figure 9.3 Standard antero-posterior X-ray with lower limbs together and in neutral rotation in child over six months.

APPLIANCES AND PLASTER CASTS USED TO MAINTAIN THE REDUCTION OF A DISLOCATED HIP

Four of the many different appliances which can be used to maintain the reduction of a dislocated hip are described below. The von Rosen and Barlow splints and the Frejka pillow are used in the management of the dislocated hip diagnosed soon after birth. The Denis Browne hip splint may be used when the diagnosis has been made either early or late. Plaster casts are used only in the later stages of management.

Splints

von Rosen splint (Rosen, 1956)
The von Rosen splint (Fig. 9.4) is H-shaped, the crossbar of the H being extended on each side. It is cut from malleable aluminium

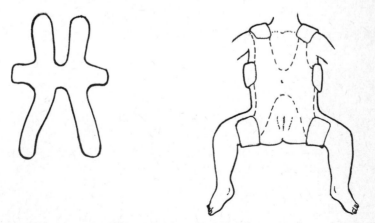

Figure 9.4 Von Rosen splint.

sheeting, padded and covered with latex rubber or plastic, the latter being less irritating to the skin of some children. Three sizes of splint are available.

APPLICATION OF THE VON ROSEN SPLINT (Fig. 9.4)
- Choose a splint of adequate size.
- Place the child supine on the splint.
- Mould the upper limbs of the splint over the shoulders, taking care that they do not press on the sides of the child's neck.
- Mould the short central limbs of the splint around the child's trunk.
- Reduce the hip and maintain the reduction by holding the hip in a position of 90 degrees of abduction/flexion, and lateral rotation. It must be possible to obtain this position easily without using force. If full abduction cannot be obtained easily, the adductors are too tight and a subcutaneous tenotomy of the adductor muscles at their origin must be performed under general anaesthesia before the splint is applied.
- Carefully mould the lower limbs of the splint around the child's thighs while keeping the hip reduced.
- Check that the hips are not flexed or abducted more than 90 degrees, and that there is not excessive tension in the adductor muscles, to avoid excessive pressure on the head of the femur and the consequent danger of epiphysitis of the femoral capital epiphysis. Barlow (1968) does not believe that there is a risk of epiphysitis occurring in the new-born. He believes that a large ossification centre in the femoral head must be present before epiphysitis can occur.
- Check that the child and especially the lower limbs do not come out of the splint when the child moves. Some movement of the hips *within* the splint is beneficial

Barlow splint (Barlow, 1962)
The Barlow splint (Fig. 9.5) consists of two strips of malleable aluminium 1 inch wide and 22 inches long (2·5 cm by 55 cm) held

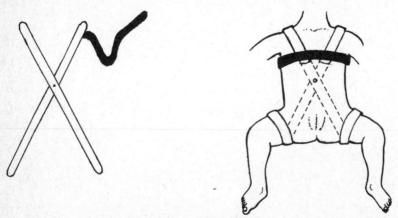

Figure 9.5   Barlow splint.

together by a single rivet 9 inches (22·5 cm) below the top end. The aluminium strips are padded on one side with felt, are covered with soft leather and are provided with a canvas strap which can be passed through slots in the top ends of the splint.

The Barlow splint is applied in a similar way to that described for the von Rosen splint. The upper ends are moulded over the shoulders where they are held together with the canvas strap which passes around the child's chest (Fig. 9.5). The lower ends of the splint are moulded around the thighs after reduction of the hip, with the hips in a position of 90 degrees of abduction/flexion and lateral rotation.

One complication of the Barlow splint is that as the two aluminium strips are joined by only a single rivet, the upper ends of the splint may press against the sides of the child's neck as the child moves.

MANAGEMENT OF A CHILD IN A SPLINT
- Instruct the mother not to take the child out of the splint. The child is tended and washed in the splint.
- Examine the child at weekly intervals, adjusting the splint as necessary.
- Replace the splint with a larger one when necessary. When a larger splint is being applied the hips must be kept in abduction, flexion and lateral rotation. This can be accomplished by lying the child on its abdomen while the splint is being changed.
- Discard the splint after twelve weeks.
- Examine the child at weekly intervals for the first six weeks after discarding the splint, then at decreasing intervals until six months have elapsed.
- X-ray the child's hips when he is six months old. If the X-ray is normal, see the child at one-yearly intervals. If the X-ray shows a difference in the acetabular angle on the affected side compared with the normal side, take further X-rays at yearly intervals until normal development of the acetabulum has occurred.

Frejka pillow (Frejka, 1954)
The Frejka pillow (Fig. 9.6) consists of a firm rectangular pad filled with feathers or kapok which may be divided transversely into three sections. Attached to the upper end of the pad are two long straps, joined in the region of the scapulae, which pass over the shoulders to be reattached by buckles to the lower end of the pad. There are two shorter straps which pass around the sides of the trunk.

APPLICATION OF THE FREJKA PILLOW (Fig. 9.6)
- Choose a suitable Frejka pillow. The width of the pad should be just less than the distance between the popliteal fossae when the hips are in a position of 90 degrees of abduction and flexion.

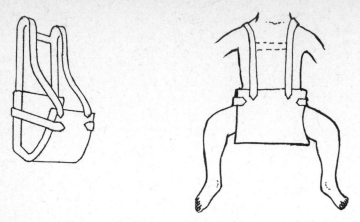

Figure 9.6   Frejka pillow.

- Lie the Frejka pillow flat on a firm surface.
- Place the child's sacrum on the upper part of the pad and then fold the pad forwards between the abducted and flexed lower limbs and up over the front of the abdomen.
- Pass the long straps over the shoulders and buckle them to the pad over the abdomen.
- Pass the short straps around the trunk and over the thighs and buckle them to the pad over the abdomen.
- Check that the pad is held firmly against the perineum.

Frejka originally introduced this appliance in 1938, and since 1946 has used it regularly as the method of choice in the treatment of children in the first year of life. He claims that the dislocated femoral head slips spontaneously and without any manipulation into the acetabulum. The disadvantage of the Frejka pillow is that it must be removed frequently to clean and bathe the child.

Denis Browne hip splint

The Denis Browne hip splint (Browne, 1948) can be used in the management of congenital dislocation of the hip when the condition has been diagnosed soon after birth, or later after the child has started to walk.

The splint (Fig. 9.7) consists of a strong metal bar to which two thigh bands are attached. The position of the thigh bands on the metal bar can be altered. The thigh bands are fastened over the child's thighs either by straps and buckles or, to prevent the mother from removing the splint, by stitching. A waterproof pad, on which the child's sacrum rests, is attached to the centre of the bar between the thigh bands. Straps pass upwards from the bar over the shoulders and back to the bar, crossing each other over the back and chest where they are stitched together. The knees are left free.

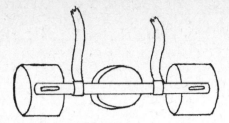

Figure 9.7 Denis Browne hip splint seen from behind.

This splint is applied in basically the same way as that described for the von Rosen and Barlow splints (Fig. 9.8).

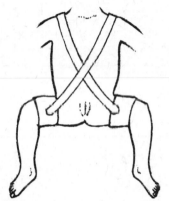

Figure 9.8 Denis Browne hip splint.

In this splint the child's hips are held in abduction/flexion and lateral rotation, the range of movement possible in each direction being about 30 degrees. The splint does not have to be removed to keep the child clean. Crawling and later walking are possible in this splint. As the child grows, the position of the thigh bands on the metal bar is adjusted. One important advantage of the splint as opposed to immobilization in a plaster cast (Lloyd-Roberts, 1971) is that it will not retain an unstable reduction as the hip re-dislocates, thus enabling the surgeon to recognise this condition early rather than late.

When used in the management of a dislocated hip diagnosed soon after birth, the splint is retained for about twelve weeks. When used on the older child, it is retained until radiological examination shows that the acetabulum is developing satisfactorily and that there is congruity of the ossifying femoral capital epiphysis in the acetabulum. This time varies between six and eighteen months. After the splint is removed, the legs slowly adduct to the neutral position during the subsequent four to six weeks. When the legs attain the neutral position a further X-ray is taken.

Plaster casts

Frog or Lorenz plaster cast

This cast (Fig. 9.9) holds the hips in a position of 90 degrees of abduction/flexion and lateral rotation as in the von Rosen, Barlow

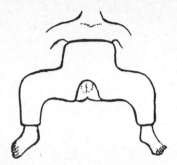

Figure 9.9   Frog or Lorenz plaster cast.

and Denis Browne splints. Unlike the splints, however, it is not generally used in the management of the dislocated hip in the newborn. The cast extends from the nipple line down to the ankles on both sides, leaving the ankles and feet free. Particular care must be taken to ensure that the cast is strong enough over the groins and buttocks. If it is not, the cast easily cracks due to the stresses imposed upon it by the strong movements of the child's limbs. An adequate opening must be allowed around the perineum to enable the child to be kept clean.

Important:
● Check that the adductor muscles of the hips are not tight and that the hips can be placed easily in the desired position before applying the cast. If the adductor muscles are tight, subcutaneous tenotomy of them at their origin must be carried out.
● Never abduct or flex the hips beyond 90 degrees as this may obstruct the blood supply to the femoral head causing ischaemia and epiphysitis even in a normal hip.

Batchelor plasters

Batchelor plasters hold the hips in abduction and medial rotation. They encircle the lower limbs only and extend from the groins to the ankles being joined by a crossbar (Fig. 9.10). The knees must be held in 15 to 20 degrees of flexion to prevent rotation of the limbs within the plaster casts.

A possible complication of the use of Batchelor plasters is an increase in the degree of anteversion of the femoral necks (Wilkinson, 1963), which may have to be corrected subsequently by derotation osteotomies of the upper ends of the femora.

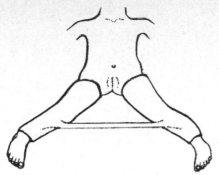

Figure 9.10   Batchelor plasters.

REFERENCES

ANDRÉN, L. and ROSEN, S. VON (1958) The diagnosis of dislocation of the hip in newborns and the primary results of immediate treatment. *Acta Radiologica*, **49**, 89.

BARLOW, T. G. (1962) Early diagnosis and treatment of congenital dislocation of hip. *Journal of Bone and Joint Surgery*, **44-B**, 292.

BARLOW, T. G. (1968) Congenital dislocation of the hip. *Hospital Medicine 2*, 571

BROWNE, D. (1948) The treatment of congenital dislocation of the hip. *Proceedings of the Royal Society of Medicine*, **41**, 388.

FREJKA, M. B. (1954) *The Danger of Conservative Treatment of Congenital Dislocation of the Hip*, p. 573. Sixth International Congress Société Internationale de Chirurgie Orthopédique et de Traumatologie.

LLOYD-ROBERTS, G. C. (1971) *Orthopaedics in Infancy and Childhood*, p. 218. London: Butterworth.

NELSON, M. A. (1966) Early diagnosis of congenital dislocation of the hip. *Journal of Bone and Joint Surgery*, **48-B**, 388.

ORTOLANI, M. (1948) *La Lussazione Congenita Dell'anca. Nuovi Criteri Diagnostici e Profilattico-Correttivi.* p. 19, Figs. 1-4; p. 20, Figs. 5 and 6 and p. 21, Fig. 7. Bologna: F. Cappelli.

ROSEN, S. VON (1956) Early diagnosis and treatment of congenital dislocation of the hip joint. *Acta Orthopaedica Scandinavica*, **26**, 136.

ROSEN, S. VON (1962) Diagnosis and treatment of congenital dislocation of the hip joint in the new-born. *Journal of Bone and Joint Surgery*, **44-B**, 284.

WILKINSON, J. A. (1963) Prime factors in the aetiology of congenital dislocation of the hip. *Journal of Bone and Joint Surgery*, **45-B**, 268.

WYNNE-DAVIES, R. (1970) Acetabular dysplasia and familial joint laxity: two aetiological factors in congenital dislocation of the hip. *Journal of Bone and Joint Surgery*, **52-B**, 704.

10. Lower limb bracing

A caliper is an external supporting device for the lower limb which may be used permanently or for a short time only. The functions of a caliper are:

To provide stability for a weakened, paralysed or unstable limb.
To relieve weight bearing.
To relieve pain.
To control deformity aggravated by postural forces.
To restrict movement of the joints of the lower limb.

Two or more of these functions may be combined. The ultimate aim is to enable the patient to walk. To achieve this a caliper must be strong, light and easy to apply and manipulate. In general the more simple an appliance is, the better.

There are two main types of caliper:

WEIGHT-RELIEVING CALIPER

The body weight is transmitted from the ischial tuberosity to a padded ring or moulded leather (bucket) top, through metal side bars to the shoe and hence the ground. In practice a weight-relieving caliper provides only partial weight relief. Its use is indicated when control of rotation of the lower limb is lost or when it is advisable to decrease the amount of body weight taken through the bones of the lower limb.

CHECKING A WEIGHT-RELIEVING CALIPER
This may be carried out in two ways.
- With the patient supine, lift the splinted leg at right angles to the body. Place the finger between the bearing point of the caliper and the ischial tuberosity. Lower the leg. If the finger is trapped, the length of the caliper is correct. If the finger can easily be removed, the caliper is too short; if the ring slips past the finger, the caliper is too long.
- With the patient standing and sitting back on the caliper top, it should just be possible to slip a finger under the patient's heel.

Advise the patient to sit back on the top of the caliper and to avoid leaning forward with the hip flexed, because as the hip is flexed, the point of contact is transferred forwards progressively from the ischial tuberosity to the ischial ramus and finally the pubic ramus (Young, 1929).

NON WEIGHT-RELIEVING CALIPER

1. Long leg brace similar in design to a weight-relieving caliper but the body weight is *not* supported on a ring. The ring merely locates the upper end of the side bars. This type of caliper is used mainly to control deformity or to restrict the movement of the joints of the lower limb.
2. Below-knee appliance, used when the ankle or foot alone requires to be controlled.

The basic design of a caliper—two metal side bars connected superiorly by a band encircling the upper thigh, and inferiorly to a shoe—may be modified, depending upon the function required of the caliper. The common variations of each part of a caliper and their functions are described below.

UPPER END OF A CALIPER

The upper end of a caliper may be fitted with a ring, cuff or block leather bucket top.

Ring top

A ring top (Fig. 10.1) consists of a metal ring padded with felt and covered with leather. It may or may not be weight-relieving. If the ring top is to transmit body weight, it must be a snug fit, otherwise the ischial tuberosity will slide through the ring, weight relief will be lost and the ring will press into the perineum where it may cause a pressure sore.

This type of top is often used on calipers for children, or for temporary calipers for adults. It is simple and cheap to construct.

Cuff top

A cuff top (Fig. 10.2) consists of a broad posterior metal thigh band padded with felt and covered with leather. Anteriorly there is a broad soft leather band adjustable by means of a strap and buckle or a Velcro fastening. A cuff top cannot be weight-relieving.

It is simple and cheap to construct, is less bulky than a ring top, and is easy to apply. A cuff top is particularly indicated when, in the presence of marked wasting of the thigh, it would be impossible to pass a ring top of the correct size over the foot or the knee.

Block leather bucket top

This type of top is made by moulding leather over a plaster cast of the thigh. The leather bucket fits accurately around the upper third of the thigh, and has a posterior curved lip on which the

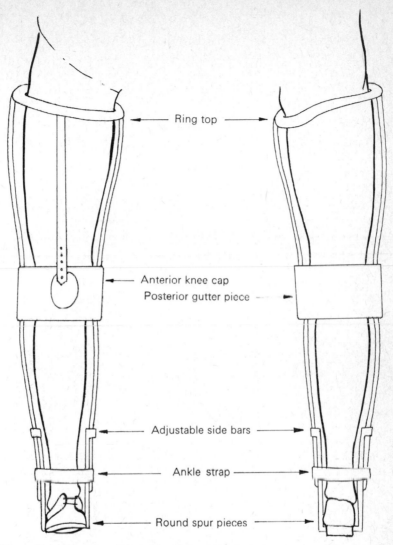

Ring top

Anterior knee cap
Posterior gutter piece

Adjustable side bars

Ankle strap

Round spur pieces

Figure 10.1   Ring top caliper with unjointed adjustable side bars, round spur pieces, anterior knee cap, posterior gutter piece and ankle strap.

ischial tuberosity rests. It is reinforced posteriorly by a transverse metal band connected to the side bars. A metal strip with a flange projects upwards to support the bucket under the ischial tuberosity. Straps and buckles or lace eyelets are fitted anteriorly (Fig. 10.3).

As this type of top must be made carefully, it is more expensive to manufacture than the other two types. Its use is reserved usually for permanent adult weight-relieving calipers. When the knee is unstable, support can be provided by extending the bucket top downwards to enclose almost the whole thigh.

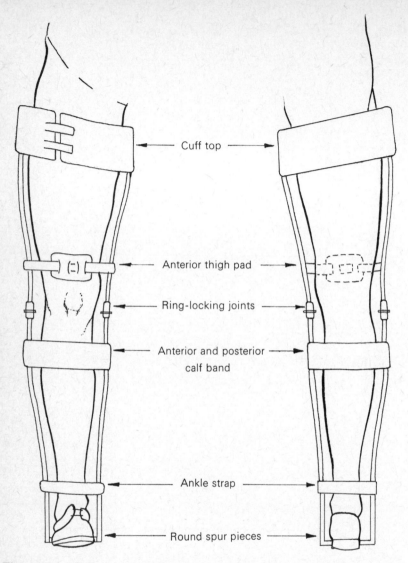

Figure 10.2   Cuff top caliper with non-adjustable side bars, ring-locking knee joints, round spur pieces, anterior thigh pad, anterior and posterior calf bands and ankle strap.

PELVIC BAND AND HIP JOINTS

A pelvic band is a padded rigid metal band covered with leather which encircles the pelvis posteriorly (extending between the anterior superior iliac spines), and presses on the sacrum. It is fastened anteriorly with a broad padded leather strap and buckle. Lateral metal bands extending downwards from the pelvic band hinge with

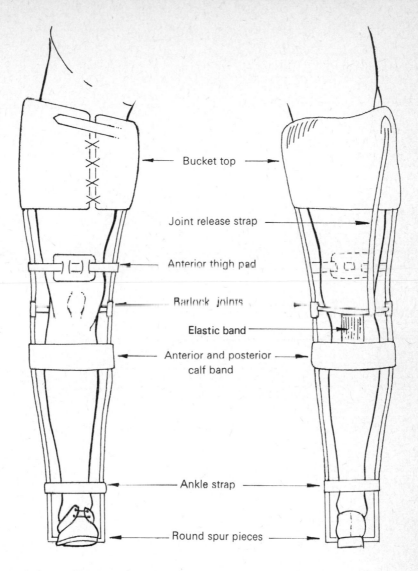

Bucket top

Joint release strap

Anterior thigh pad

Barlock joints

Elastic band

Anterior and posterior calf band

Ankle strap

Round spur pieces

Figure 10.3 Moulded leather bucket top caliper with non-adjustable side bars, barlock knee joints, round spur pieces, anterior thigh pad, anterior and posterior calf bands and ankle strap.

upward extensions of the lateral side bars of long leg calipers at the level of the hips (Fig. 10.4). It is better to use two long leg calipers with a pelvic band. If only one caliper is used, the pelvic band can rotate on the pelvis.

The hinge or hip joint may allow either free flexion or extension, or be fitted with a lock to limit these movements either separately or in combination. It is important that the hip joints of the appliance are positioned on the axis of hip flexion—parallel and

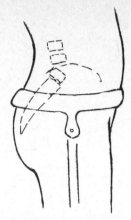

Figure 10.4   Pelvic band and hip joint. Note that the pelvic band encircles the pelvis below the anterior superior iliac spines, and the hip joint is positioned slightly in front of the greater trochanter.

adjacent to the greater trochanters of the femora—otherwise discomfort is experienced by the patient, and unnecessary stress is thrown upon the appliance. A limited abduction joint may be needed also for the older, heavier child or adult to prevent the rapid wearing out of the flexion-extension joint.

If support to decrease lumbar lordosis is required upward extensions from the pelvic band to a lumbo-sacral support may be added.

The function of a pelvic band with hip joints is to prevent the development of a flexion deformity and to control adduction and medial rotation at the hip, in the presence of muscle imbalance around the hip, following anterior poliomyelitis, spina bifida or cerebral palsy. In addition these appliances increase the stability of the spine.

These appliances are always very cumbersome, even although they can be made with only a lateral side bar to the long leg calipers when the pelvic band is well fitting. They should be recommended only after very careful consideration, as the patients who require such appliances are seldom able to walk more than a few yards, even although their stability and mobility may be improved. Light appliances which simply brace the lower limbs may be better, the patient using crutches and a swinging gait.

SIDE BARS

Stability is provided by metal side bars which must be both strong and light. Steel is used for calipers for the lower limbs in heavy patients, the active child, and when severe spasticity or athetosis is present, and for permanent calipers. Duralumin is suitable for the side bars of light appliances. The moving parts, joints and the attachments of the caliper to the shoe, are always made of steel.

The side bars are shaped to the contour of the limb and must not rub the skin. In children they must be adjustable for length to allow for growth (Fig. 10.1).

The side bars are attached proximally to the ring, cuff or block leather bucket top, and distally are slotted into the heel of the shoe or boot. Knee joints may be incorporated.

KNEE JOINTS

The normal knee is a combination of a hinge and a sliding joint. It is not practicable to make an artificial joint which accurately follows normal knee movement. The nearest point corresponding to the natural axis of movement is situated $\frac{1}{2}$ inch (1·25 cm) above the joint line, and a little posterior to its centre.

Ring lock knee joint

The ring lock knee joint is the safest and most durable. It is illustrated in Figures 10.2 and 10.5. The axis of rotation of the joint is eccentric to prevent the anterior edge of the male section from projecting when the joint is flexed. The ring is pulled up to allow the knee to flex and is pushed downwards when the knee is extended, to lock the hinge. A spring-loaded ball controls the position of the ring. A patient must have sufficient power in the fingers to manipulate the ring lock. In hemiplegia, the ring lock knee joint must be fitted to the same side of the caliper as the *normal*

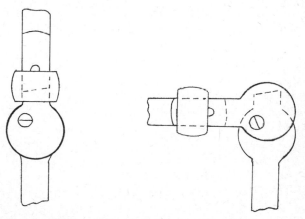

Figure 10.5   Manual ring-lock knee joint.

upper limb, and a simple non-locking joint to the other side bar.

Ring lock knee joints with springs which automatically lock the joint when the knee is extended, may be fitted. An *automatic ring lock* must not be fitted to all four hinges when two calipers are worn, as it is impossible for a patient to manipulate all four ring locks simultaneously while attempting to sit down. A further modification of the automatic ring lock is called the *rod-spring ring lock*. This consists of a ring lock to the ring of which a length of rod with a co-axial spring is fitted. An upward pull on the rod raises the ring and frees the joint. When the knee is extended, release of the rod allows the co-axial spring to push the ring down and lock the joint. This type of locking knee joint is used when a patient is unable to lean forward far enough to operate an ordinary ring lock knee joint, or when he cannot regain the erect position after bending forward.

Barlock (Swiss lock) knee joint

The barlock type of knee joint (Figs. 10.3 and 10.6) locks automatically on extension of the knee. By pulling on a strap attached

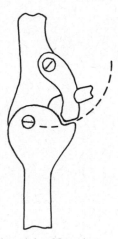

Figure 10.6   Barlock knee joint. Note the arc of movement of the pawl.

to a curved posterior bar connecting the pawls, the pawls on both sides are released simultaneously, thus allowing knee flexion. The release strap from the curved bar is attached to the top, outer edge of the block leather bucket or ring top. A broad elastic band connecting the curved bar to the calf band provides the necessary tension for the locking device (Fig. 10.3).

The main disadvantage of this type of locking knee joint is that with lateral malalignment, the pawls may not fit into their notches accurately, and therfore malfunction may occur. This joint is used only on permanent appliances for patients who will always have to walk with an extended knee, as this joint cannot be left unlocked. The barlock knee joint must never be used when spasticity is present, as failure is very likely to occur.

It is important that this type of knee joint is manufactured correctly. The tips of the pawls move through an arc of a circle. To ensure accurate locking, the lugs on the distal side of the knee joint must lie on the same arc, and must therefore point upwards and backwards (Fig. 10.6).

Posterior off-set knee joint (Fig. 10.7)

The posterior off-set knee joint is a non-locking type of joint. When incorporated into a long leg caliper, the axis of movement of the joint is situated posterior to the axis of flexion/extension of the knee. This means that when the knee is in at least 10 degrees of hyperextension, the posterior off-set knee joint is stable as the body weight passes down a line anterior to the axis of movement of the joint.

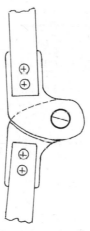

Figure 10.7   Posterior off-set knee joint.

These types of knee joints are used instead of locking knee joints in the 'cosmetic' appliances, which have been introduced recently, for patients with a flail lower limb who exhibit at least 10 degrees of hyperextension at the knee (see later). Hyperextension can be aided if necessary by lowering the heel of the shoe slightly and adding a small raise to the sole.

Knee joints usually are not fitted to children's calipers. Locking knee joints may be essential for a spastic child or to aid in sitting at school. They are reserved for permanent adult calipers, either weight relieving or non-weight relieving, to ease sitting.

HEEL ATTACHMENT OF SIDE BARS

The distal ends of a caliper may be attached to the shoe or boot by means of heel sockets or via a stirrup.

Heel sockets

The distal ends of the side bars of a caliper are bent inwards at a right angle and slotted into metal sockets fitted into the heel of the shoe. The caliper ends (spur pieces) and the heel sockets may be round or flat (rectangular).

Round sockets are employed when muscle control is adequate and the patient is able to dorsiflex and plantar-flex his ankle. The disadvantages of the round socket are that movement at the anatomical ankle joint does not correspond with the level of the ankle joint of the appliance, with the result that the appliance rides up and down with dorsiflexion and plantar-flexion; compression of the calf by the calf band occurs on dorsiflexion; and the heel tends to slip out of the shoe. The advantages of round sockets are that they are easier to make and adjust, the apparatus is lighter, and different shoes are interchangeable easily.

Round sockets are used usually for children's calipers, and for temporary calipers for adults.

Flat (or rectangular) sockets. This type of heel socket allows easy interchangeability of shoes but does not allow the heel of the shoe to pivot. It is therefore usually employed with an ankle hinge (Fig. 10.12). A flail ankle could be controlled by flat sockets without an ankle hinge, but fixation is too rigid and the shoe would not withstand the strain unless it was reinforced. Flat sockets are expensive and are reserved usually for permanent calipers.

Stirrups

There are two types of stirrup attachment, the ordinary stirrup and the sandal or insert stirrup.

Ordinary stirrup. An ordinary stirrup consists of a U-shaped piece of metal which is rigidly fixed to the anterior part of the underside of the heel of the shoe. The arms of the U pass up and slightly backwards (about 5 to 6 degrees) on each side of the shoe to ankle joints positioned on the axis of movement of the anatomical ankle joint.

Sandal or insert type of stirrup. In this type a footplate is attached to the stirrup, both of which are placed inside the shoe (Fig. 10.8). The main advantage of this method is that shoes can be changed easily. Moreover, as the foot plate and stirrup take up room in the shoe, it may be possible to wear shoes of the same

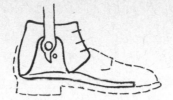

Figure 10.8   Sandal or insert type of stirrup.

size when there is a discrepancy in the size of the feet, as may occur in patients who have had poliomyelitis. The disadvantages of the sandal type of stirrup are that pressure sores may develop, and control of movement between the foot and the foot plate is difficult. The sandal type of stirrup must never be used for patients with paraplegia or sensory disturbance in the foot.

Toe-out

When arranging the attachment of the side bars of a caliper to a shoe by any of the above methods, it is necessary to provide toe-out, to prevent the patient from tripping over his toes. The amount of toe-out required is determined individually. It depends upon the relationship between the axes of movement of the knee and ankle joints, which in turn depends upon the degree of tibial torsion present. The amount of toe-out usually provided is 10 to 15 degrees. To achieve this the attachment of the inner side bar of the caliper is positioned slightly posterior to that of the outer side bar (Fig. 10.9).

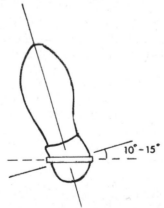

Figure 10.9   Toe-out.

ANKLE JOINTS

A joint at the level of the ankle follows the natural ankle movement. It can be constructed to allow free movement, or to limit plantar-flexion or dorsiflexion or both.

It is essential that the axes of movement of the mechanical and anatomical ankle joints are identical. The axis of anatomical movement lies on a line which passes from just below the tip of the medial malleolus and which bisects the lateral malleolus one half inch above its tip.

When ankle joints are incorporated in a caliper, flat heel sockets (Fig. 10.12) or a stirrup are necessary. As these fittings are difficult and expensive to make, they are reserved usually for permanent adult calipers or when a toe raising device is required.

CONTROL OF ANKLE JOINT MOVEMENT

Movement at the anatomical ankle joint can be controlled by specially constructed mechanical ankle joints, or, when round heel sockets are used, by heel stops.

A *heel stop* is a metal lug attached to the anterior or posterior aspects of a round heel socket (Fig. 10.10), to limit dorsiflexion or

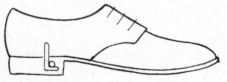

Figure 10.10 Back heel stop fitted to a round heel socket to control plantar-flexion at the ankle joint.

plantar-flexion respectively. If plantar-flexion is weak, excessive dorsiflexion can be controlled with a front or calcaneus stop. Conversely if dorsiflexion is weak, foot control can be improved by adding a back or equinus stop. In the presence of a flail ankle, front and back stops can be fitted so that only a few degrees of dorsiflexion and plantar-flexion are possible. The main disadvantage of this method of controlling ankle movement is that the axis of movement of the appliance does not correspond with that of the ankle joint, with the result that considerable stress is imposed upon the heel sockets and the shoe itself.

TOE-RAISING DEVICES

When weakness of dorsiflexion is present, the fitting of a device to aid dorsiflexion will improve greatly the patient's function. Tripping over uneven ground and the characteristic high stepping gait will be abolished. As stated above, the fitting of a back stop or a mechanical ankle joint constructed to control plantar-flexion will passively control a drop foot. There are however a number of active methods employed which utilise a spring device of some sort.

Double below-knee iron, round heel sockets and toe-raising spring

The simplest type of toe-raising spring is illustrated in Figure 10.11. The spring is attached to the double below-knee iron which fits into round heel sockets, by a Y-shaped strap. The lower end of the spring is attached to the middle of the dorsum of the shoe, at

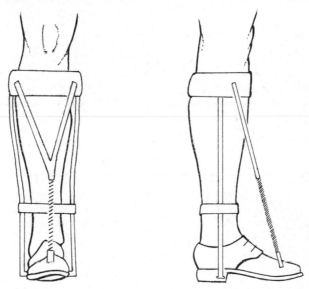

Figure 10.11 Double below-knee iron, round spur pieces, toe-raising spring and ankle strap.

the level of the metatarso-phalangeal joints, by a small leather lug stitched to the shoe. This is a cheap and effective mechanism but it is obvious, especially when worn by women, and considerable stress is imposed upon the heel sockets and the shoe.

Double below-knee iron, ankle joints, flat heel sockets and toe-raising spring

A less obvious toe-raising spring is that employed with an ankle joint and flat spur pieces and heel sockets as illustrated in Figure 10.12. The spring is attached to the outer side bar (or both side bars) of a caliper or double below-knee iron by an adjustable strap and buckle or wire rod, and to a lug projecting forward from the centre of the ankle joint. This apparatus is heavy and expensive. Considerable stress is still imposed upon the shoe and heel sockets, and with time the flat spur pieces become worn and loose.

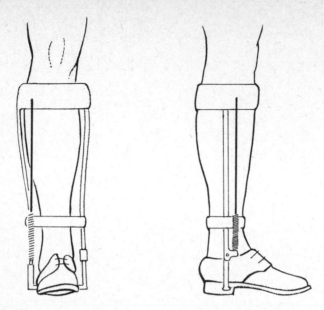

Figure 10.12   Double below-knee iron with ankle joints, flat spur pieces, toe-raising spring and ankle strap.

Double below-knee iron with rubber torsion socket

When the force required to overcome the drop foot is not great, a toe-raising device concealed in the heel can be used. Originally this device consisted of a number of turns of spring piano wire wound round a rod (Tuck, 1957). Square sockets were sunk in each end of the rod to take the spur pieces. A similar toe-raising mechanism with a rubber bush vulcanised to the rod is now available (Tuck, 1962). The spring action results from torsional stresses in the rubber which can be varied by a screw thread. The disadvantages of the rubber bush are that it may rapidly wear out and it can be fitted only to a broad-heeled shoe. Both these devices are light and cheap, the later type being mass produced.

Exeter coil spring toe-raising appliance

For children under the age of five years, a below-knee appliance fitted with a toe-raising spring, even if made of Duralumin, would be too heavy. In such cases an Exeter coil spring toe-raising appliance (Fig. 10.13) which combines the functions of supporting side bars and a toe-raising spring in a simple light appliance, can be used. This appliance, however, is very restrictive, with the result that the attachment of the spring steel to the heel of the shoe may become loose, or the steel itself may break.

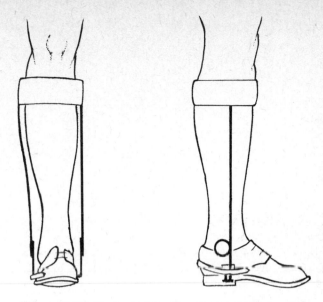

Figure 10.13   Exeter double coil-spring toe-raising appliance.

Ortholene★ drop foot splint (Fig. 10.14)

When the ankle joint can be dorsiflexed passively to at least a right angle, and when spasticity is absent, an Ortholene★ or Perplas★ (both are high-density polyethylenes) drop foot splint can be prescribed.

From a plaster-of-Paris cast of the leg, taken with the ankle held above a right angle if possible, a positive cast is made, over which a strip of high-density polyethylene is moulded. This strip extends downwards from behind the upper calf, around the heel and forwards under the sole to the base of the toes. When the high-density polyethylene has cooled, it is trimmed to ensure a snug fit inside the shoe, and the edges are chamfered, especially under the toes. If necessary a calf pad of Plastazote can be added to improve the cosmetic appearance of the leg.

The splint is worn next to the skin. A Velcro strap may be fitted to the upper end to keep it closely applied to the back of the calf, or an elastic stocking may be worn.

This splint overcomes the cosmetic and mechanical disadvantages of the previously described appliances. In addition it overcomes the disadvantage of some of the present-day commercial footwear, the heels of which are hollow plastic mouldings unsuitable for the insertion of heel sockets.

★ See Appendix.

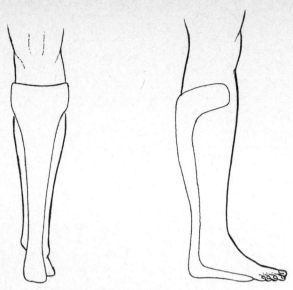

Figure 10.14   Ortholene drop foot splint.

T-STRAPS

A T-strap is cut from leather. The vertical limb of the T is attached
to the shoe at the junction of the upper with the sole. It is placed
well forward. The strap is cut with long tongues so that the upper
end of the strap encircles both the ankle and the side bar with the

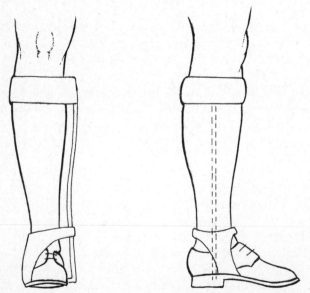

Figure 10.15   Single inside below-knee iron with round spur piece and outside
T-strap.

buckle on the other side of the leg, and the end of the strap pointing backwards.

A T-strap may be attached to either the inside or the outside of the shoe, to provide stability and to substitute for paralysed or partially paralysed invertor or evertor muscles. A single below-knee appliance (side bar) is used in conjunction with a T-strap (Fig. 10.15).

Examples:

1. When the tibialis anterior and tibialis posterior muscles are weak, but the peroneal muscles are strong, the foot will assume a position of valgus. This deformity can be controlled by an outside iron and an inside T-strap.
2. A varus deformity from weakness of the peroneal muscles can be controlled with an inside iron and an outside T-strap.

RETAINING STRAPS AND BANDS

In addition to the above modifications which may be made to a caliper, it must be remembered that the limb must be retained within the caliper. This is achieved by using various leather straps and bands. These are described below.

ANKLE STRAP. The spur pieces of an appliance must be retained in the heel sockets. A T-strap will perform this function as well as correcting a varus or valgus deformity. In the absence of a T-strap, an ankle strap must be present. An ankle strap is attached to the outer side bar, passes around the inner side bar and lower part of the leg, and back to the outer side bar where it is buckled firmly. (Figs. 10.1, 10.2, 10.3, 10.11, 10.12, and 10.17.)

CALF BAND and ANTERIOR THIGH PAD. When a knee joint is used a calf band and an anterior thigh pad are fitted. The calf band, lined with felt and covered with leather, is attached to the side bars just below the knee joint. A padded anterior thigh pad is fitted above the knee joint (Figs. 10.2 and 10.3). It is not required when a long leather bucket top is used. The calf band and the anterior thigh pad are fastened with a strap and buckle or a Velcro fastening. Eyelets and a lace can also be used for the latter.

KNEE PAD. A knee pad is not always fitted to hinged calipers as it limits knee flexion. Its function is to stabilise the knee in a non-hinged caliper. In addition to the anterior knee pad, a leather gutter piece is attached to the side bars to lie across the popliteal fossa (Fig. 10.1).

A knee pad can also be used to control or to prevent the development of a valgus or varus deformity of the knee in the presence of ligamentous laxity. To control a valgus deformity of the

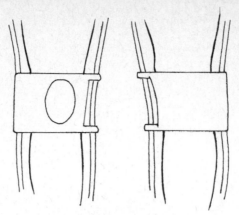

Figure 10.16   Knock-knee pad.

knee, the pad is attached to the outer side bar and passes around the knee (between the knee and the inner side bar) to be attached again to the outer side bar. In addition there are two narrow straps which attach the top and bottom of the knee pad loosely to the inner side bar, to control knee flexion (Fig. 10.16). To control a varus deformity of the knee, the attachments of the knee pad are reversed.

PATTEN-ENDED CALIPER

When it is essential for a limb to be relieved of all weight bearing, a patten-ended caliper (Fig. 10.17) is required. This type of caliper was commonly used in the ambulant treatment of Perthes' disease of the hip. It is used less often for this purpose today.

A patten-ended caliper has a snugly fitting ring top. The steel side bars, without knee joints, are adjustable for length and are prolonged about 3 inches (7·6 cm) below the heel. The distal ends of the side bars are welded to a steel ring, the patten, from which a strap passes to the back of the shoe, to control plantar-flexion of the ankle. The foot of the affected leg is thus kept sufficiently clear of the ground to prevent the child from taking weight on his toes. In addition posterior thigh and calf bands, a knee pad and an ankle strap are provided.

Normal footwear is worn on the affected side, but a compensating patten must be added to the opposite shoe to accommodate the increase in length of the affected lower limb (Fig. 10.18).

The length of the caliper must be adjusted repeatedly to allow for growth, otherwise the child will soon bear weight on its toes. Whether or not this is occurring can be determined by examining the toe of the shoe worn on the affected side, for the presence of wear.

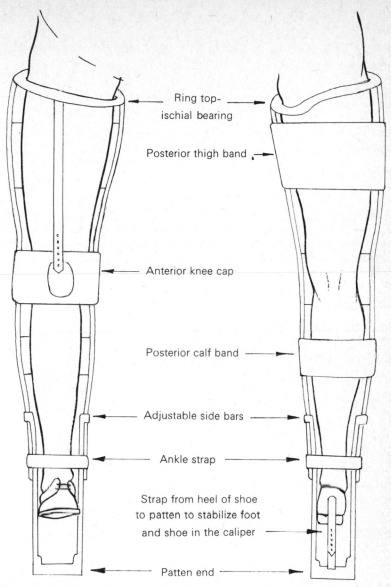

Ring top-
ischial bearing

Posterior thigh band

Anterior knee cap

Posterior calf band

Adjustable side bars

Ankle strap

Strap from heel of shoe
to patten to stabilize foot
and shoe in the caliper

Patten end

Figure 10.17 Patten ended caliper with ischial bearing ring top, adjustable side bars, posterior thigh band, anterior knee cap, posterior calf band, ankle strap and strap from heel of shoe to patten.

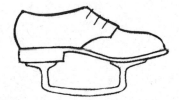

Figure 10.18 Compensatory patten on a normal shoe.

THE 'COSMETIC' LONG LEG CALIPER (Fig. 10.19)

The long leg calipers illustrated in Figures 10.1, 10.2, and 10.3 have a number of disadvantages. They are cumbersome, heavy, rigid and often uncomfortable. They frequently break, are not cosmetically acceptable especially to women, and take many hours to make. In addition all the patient's shoes have to be fitted with heel sockets, and as the foot of the affected limb is often smaller, the patient may have to buy two pairs of shoes each time.

To overcome these inherent disadvantages and the additional problem of the unsuitable present-day commercial footwear, a new type of long leg caliper for use in cases of flaccid paralysis of the lower limb has been developed by Mr W. H. Tuck at The Royal National Orthopaedic Hospital. This development has resulted from the introduction of plastics and has received additional impetus from the previous development of the Ortholene drop foot splint.

This new appliance is fitted with a bucket top made from high-density polyethylene moulded around a positive cast of the upper thigh and ischial region. Where the shape and size of the foot will

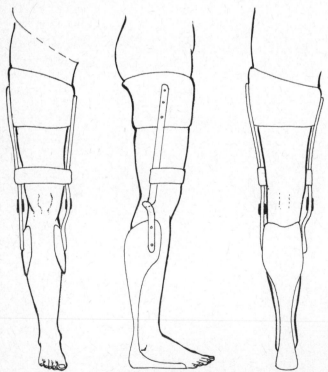

Figure 10.19 'Cosmetic' long leg caliper. Note that the side bars end just below the knee where they are riveted to an Ortholene drop foot splint. Posterior off-set knee joints are illustrated.

allow, the bucket top is riveted, forming a rigid cylinder which is threaded over the limb when the caliper is applied.

The side bars terminate just below the knee where they are riveted to a modified Ortholene drop foot splint. This results in the caliper being lighter, and more resilient and cosmetically acceptable to the patient. The cosmetic appearance can be improved further by adding a false calf of Plastazote. The side bars are finished by sand blasting and then heat-coated with nylon.

Ring-lock knee joints (Fig. 10.5) are used commonly, barlock joints only rarely. When at least 10 degrees of hyperextension is present at the knee, posterior off-set knee joints (Fig. 10.7) can be fitted instead of locking knee joints, providing that the patient's other limb is normal, as the patient's stability depends upon his being able to maintain hyperextension at the knee.

The caliper, with the addition of a knee or anterior thigh pad and possibly an anterior calf band, is worn next to the skin in the same way as the Ortholene drop-foot splint.

The choice of suitable footwear is wide. The heel must be broad and it is advisable that it should not exceed 1 to 1·5 inches (2·5 to 3·75 cm) in height. As the caliper fits inside the shoe, compensation can be made easily for any discrepancy in size of the feet.

These new types of calipers have a number of advantages over the older types. They are much lighter, weighing about half that of the older calipers; they are cosmetically acceptable; they allow movement of the foot and caliper within the shoe which results in the patient being better able to adapt to uneven surfaces; they are more hygienic; they are quicker to make, the time being reduced by about one-third; and they are no more expensive.

Appliances of similar design (Hartshill lower limb appliances, Yates, 1968) but using polypropylene instead of Ortholene* or Perplas* are made by Salt & Son Ltd.*

CARE OF CALIPERS

Every patient who wears a caliper must be instructed in its care, and must be advised to—

- Always handle the caliper with care, and to avoid dropping it.
- Examine his skin every night for evidence of undue pressure from the caliper.
- Each week open all locks and remove any accumulated dirt or fluff.
- Oil each joint weekly.
- Inspect all moving parts for wear, and ensure that all bolts and screws are present and not loose.
- Inspect all leather parts regularly, keep them in good condition, and get any necessary repairs carried out immediately.
- Keep the heels and the soles of the footwear in good condition.

* See Appendix.

PRESCRIBING A LOWER LIMB APPLIANCE

The main functions of the lower limbs are support of the trunk and propulsion. The aim of prescribing appliances for the lower limbs is to improve these functions by providing stability, overcoming weakness, relieving pain and controlling deformities. To achieve this the appliance must be as strong, light, simple and easy to apply and manipulate as possible, and in addition it should be cosmetically acceptable to the patient.

Before an appliance is prescribed, careful evaluation of existing function and examination of the affected limb or limbs must be carried out. The problem and its possible solution must be discussed with the patient and the appliance maker (Orthotist). Occasionally operations are necessary to correct deformities, in order to simplify the manufacture and fitting of an appliance.

When an appliance is prescribed, all the relevant personal details of the patient, the diagnosis, the part to be braced, the type of appliance, its intended function and the details of its composition must be entered on the prescription.

Sample prescription

A child contracted poliomyelitis which affected one of his lower limbs, leaving weakness particularly of extension of the knee and dorsiflexion of the ankle. Contractures of the joints have not developed.

Name : JOHN SMITH.

Age : 13 years.

Diagnosis : Poliomyelitis right lower limb with weakness of the quadriceps and dorsiflexors of the ankle.

Caliper required to stabilise the knee and compensate for weakness of dorsiflexion of the ankle.

Rx. : Right long leg caliper with cuff top, adjustable side bars, double automatic ring lock knee joints, round spur pieces and heel sockets with posterior heel stops, anterior thigh pad, calf band and ankle strap.

REFERENCES

Tuck, W. H. (1957) Drop-foot appliance with concealed spring. *Journal of Bone and Joint Surgery*, **39-B**, 335.

Tuck, W. H. (1962) Drop-foot appliance with rubber torsion socket. *Journal of Bone and Joint Surgery*, **44-B**, 896.

Yates, G. (1968) A method for the provision of lightweight aesthetic orthopaedic appliances. *Orthopaedics*, Oxford, **1**, 153.

Young, C. S. (1929) A study in fitting the ring of the Thomas splint. *Journal of the American Medical Association*, **93**, 602.

11. Footwear

The manufacture of special footwear, or alterations or additions to existing footwear, may be necessary to accommodate deformed feet, to relieve pain, or to compensate for shortening of a lower limb.

SURGICAL FOOTWEAR

Any attempt to accommodate severely deformed feet within normal footwear will result in pain, callosity and bursa formation, and occasionally skin ulceration, from localised areas of excessive pressure. These complications can be avoided by wearing surgical footwear made on a last constructed from accurate measurements or from a plaster cast of the deformed feet.

When a foot is deformed, for example by hammer toes or hallux valgus, but is still plantigrade, careful measurements of the foot are adequate for the construction of the last. When the abnormality of the foot is such that the plantar surface of the foot cannot be accommodated on a leather sole, for example severe untreated talipes equino-varus, a preliminary plaster cast of the foot is essential. An inside cork sole shaped to the contour of the base of the foot is made. This ensures that the body weight is transmitted evenly over a large surface area, thus avoiding localised areas of excessive pressure.

Shoes are usually prescribed when the deformity is limited to the forefoot, and boots if the foot is grossly deformed, if the hind foot is involved, if scars are present around the ankle which would be rubbed by the top of the shoe, or if a large raise is required. The toe of the shoes or boots supplied is commonly plain because it has a smooth inner surface.

When surgical footwear is prescribed, consideration must also be given to the size of the opening through which the foot is to be inserted, and the method of fastening to be employed. For example a rigid or flail foot requires a large opening such as is provided with the Canadian open pattern footwear, or with lacing extended distally to the toe.

Patients who have limited finger function, such as may occur in rheumatoid arthritis, may be unable to manage laces and may therefore require footwear of the slip-on variety. This may also apply to patients with poor hip flexion who are unable to reach shoe laces. The replacement of ordinary shoe laces with elastic laces can be of great help in the latter situation.

Most surgical footwear is still made of leather, but the hand-sewn welted leather sole is gradually being replaced by the micro-cellular (rubber) sole which is cemented to the upper. A microcellular sole and heel is lighter, more flexible and harder wearing than leather.

Over the last few years many new synthetic materials have been developed. These are now beginning to be used in the manufacture of surgical footwear. From materials such as Plastazote* (a high-density polyethylene) covered with Yampi* (a plastic), vacuum-formed shoes and bootees can be made.

Vacuum-formed Plastazote and Yampi footwear (Tuck, 1971)

This type of footwear may be used in the conservative management of any severely deformed foot, such as may occur in rheumatoid arthritis, after partial amputation or leprosy, or when trophic ulcer-ation or gross swelling is present. Shoes or bootees can be made, the latter being prescribed when the foot is severely deformed.

A preliminary plaster-of-Paris cast of the foot is taken, from which a positive plaster cast is made. A Plastazote inner sole is initially formed, and is then added to and trimmed as necessary to obtain a flat surface. The upper is then formed, and after trimming it is attached to the inner sole with an adhesive. A microcellular sole and heel and a Velcro fixing are added finally.

This type of footwear has a number of advantages over the presently accepted surgical shoes and boots. It fits snugly around the heel and mid-foot; it provides total surface contact with the sole of the foot, thus ensuring that the body-weight is spread evenly over a large area and that localised areas of excessive pressure are avoided; it is about one-third the weight of similar leather footwear; it can be washed and is therefore more hygienic; the Velcro fixing is managed easily even by severely deformed hands; and it will last for up to twelve months. The main disadvantages are that some patients experience excessive sweating of their feet and the appearance is not so smart as that of leather footwear.

HOW TO CHECK THAT FOOTWEAR FITS CORRECTLY

The fit of any footwear is of the greatest importance during weight bearing and walking because there is a tendency for the foot to lengthen and broaden, due to the stretching of the ligaments of the foot, under the influence of body weight. Therefore the patient must be asked to stand and walk when footwear is checked.

* See Appendix.

- Excessive pressure must not be exerted on the foot by the upper or inner sole.
- There must be adequate room over the dorsum of the toes and over the sides of the heads of the first and fifth metatarsals.
- There must be a gap between the ends of all the toes and the toe of the shoe or boot.
- The patient must be able to move all his toes freely.
- The metatarso-phalangeal joint of the big toe must be level with the inner curve of the sole, where the sole starts to curve laterally under the arch.
- The upper must fit snugly around the ankle and the back of the heel.
- The waist of the shoe or boot must grip the foot firmly enough to prevent the foot from slipping forward or backward.

MODIFICATION TO EXISTING FOOTWEAR

Although surgical footwear as discussed above may be required for the management of painful feet, particularly in cases of severe deformity, much foot pain can be alleviated by prescribing various additions or modifications to existing footwear. For convenience of discussion, pain in the foot is considered to arise from one or more of the following four sites: medial longitudinal arch, metatarsal arch, heel and toes. An accurate diagnosis must be made before these additions or modifications are prescribed and it must be remembered that foot symptoms often can be relieved by physiotherapy.

Medial longitudinal arch

Pain arising from the medial longitudinal arch of the foot may be due to foot strain (from prolonged unaccustomed standing, rapid increase in body weight, resumption of weight-bearing after a long period of bed rest), or degenerative changes in the tarsal and tarso-metatarsal joints. It is usually associated with flattening of the medial longitudinal arch and can be relieved by supporting that arch. This support can be obtained in a number of different ways.

Insoles

Valgus insoles. These are constructed commonly from felt or sponge rubber covered with leather and mounted on a firm leather insole (Fig. 11.1). Occasionally rigid arch supports made from metal or plastic are prescribed.

The support extends from the middle of the heel forward under the medial longitudinal arch to half an inch (1·25 cm) behind the metatarsal heads. The height of the arch support must be correct. It must not be too high for the rigid flat foot, or too low for a mobile flat foot. Even if the condition is unilateral it is advisable to prescribe a pair of insoles.

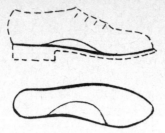

Figure 11.1 Valgus insole—full length. The support extends from the middle of the heel forwards under the medial longitudinal arch to the metatarsal heads.

When marked flattening of the medial longitudinal arch is present attention must be paid to the metatarsal arch because support for both arches may be necessary. A combined valgus and metatarsal arch support may be prescribed also for pes cavus, so that the body weight is evenly distributed and pressure on the metatarsal heads is relieved.

Insoles may be either of full or three-quarter length. A full length insole is less likely to shift within the shoe with movement of the foot. It does, however, decrease the amount of space in which the toes can move, and therefore should not be prescribed if there is any tendency to hammer toe or claw toe deformity.

As an insole takes up space within a shoe it may be necessary to advise the patient to buy footwear half a size larger than he usually wears. Patients who have been prescribed insoles should be advised to wear them initially for only a short period during the day, gradually increasing the length of time until they are wearing them continuously.

Shoe alterations

(1) *Thomas heel*. The front surface (breastline) of a normal heel is slightly concave and runs transversely across the sole. In a Thomas heel (Fig. 11.2), the medial part of the breastline is extended forward at least 1 inch (2·5 cm), at which point the front of the heel lies under the navicular bone. This gives support to the medial longitudinal arch.

(2) *Medial shank filler*. Heavy patients sometimes depress the longitudinal arch of their shoes. This can be prevented and support for the medial longitudinal arch of the foot can be obtained by adding a medial shank filler, which fills in the gap between the ground and

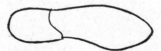

Figure 11.2 Thomas heel.

the under surface of the longitudinal arch of the shoe on the medial side. A medial shank filler extends from the medial breastline of the heel to the head of the first metatarsal where it is feathered to blend with the sole level with the break of the shoe (Fig. 11.3).

(3) *Medial heel and lateral sole wedges.* This combination of wedges (cross wedging) produces a tendency to invert the heel and to evert the forefoot, which results in elevation of the medial longitudinal arch.

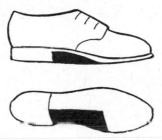

Figure 11.3   Medial shank filler.

Metatarsal arch

Pain arising from the metatarsal arch region of the foot is usually due to the prominence of one or more of the central three metatarsal heads in the sole of the foot, associated with dorsal subluxation or dislocation of the respective metatarso-phalangeal joints. A hammer or claw toe deformity is usually present also. The latter may be associated with pes cavus. Other causes of metatarsalgia are Freiberg's disease of a metatarsal head, an interdigital neuroma, March fracture or disease such as rheumatoid arthritis. Symptoms can be alleviated by relieving pressure on the plantar aspect of the metatarsal heads.

Insoles, etc.

(1) *Metatarsal arch support.* A metatarsal arch support consists of a pad of sponge rubber mounted on a firm leather insole and covered with leather. A single domed support (Fig. 11.4) will provide

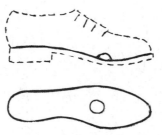

Figure 11.4   Domed metatarsal support, to relive pressure on one or two of the middle metatarsal heads.

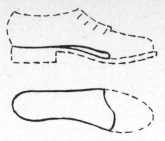

Figure 11.5   Full width, three quarter length metatarsal arch support. The support must lie behind the metatarsal heads.

support for one or two of the middle metatarsal heads. When support for more than one or two metatarsal heads is indicated, a full width arch support is prescribed (Fig. 11.5).

A valgus and metatarsal arch support can be combined on one insole. As metatarsalgia is often associated with hammer or claw toe deformities, care must be taken before prescribing a metatarsal arch support on a full length insole. In such a situation a three-quarter length insole is preferable.

(2) *Metatarsal pad and garter*. This consists of a pad of sponge rubber mounted on a broad elastic band, which is slipped over the foot (Fig. 11.6). It is useful in relieving mild metatarsalgia and has the additional advantage of allowing the patient to change his foot-wear without having to transfer any insoles.

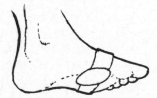

Figure 11.6   Metatarsal pad and garter.

Metatarsal arch supports must be of adequate thickness and must be positioned correctly. This is very important. *They must lie behind* (not under) *the metatarsal heads*. Pressure on the metatarsal heads is reduced by the body weight being transferred through the necks of the metatarsals.

A new metatarsal arch support must be checked after it has been worn for one or two weeks. Prominent metatarsal heads tend to wear a depression in, or leave a clearer mark upon the insole. If the arch support is in the correct position neither of these two signs will be present. If these changes are present upon the insole, then the support is placed too far posteriorly, or is not high enough, and if present upon the arch support, then the support is placed too far forwards.

Shoe alterations

Metatarsal bar. Pressure on the metatarsal heads can be relieved also by placing a raised bar of leather or microcellular rubber across the sole of the shoe directly behind and parallel to the line between the first and fifth metatarsal heads (Fig. 11.7). The anterior and posterior extensions of the bar are feathered into the sole. The bar takes the body weight behind the metatarsal heads and provides a rocker movement. The average height of the bar for adults is 5/8ths of an inch (1·6 cm). The disadvantage of this method is that the useful life of the bar is short due to wear, but it can be renewed easily without damage to the shoe.

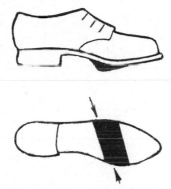

Figure 11.7 Metatarsal bar for metatarsalgia. Note that the apex of the bar lies immediately behind and parallel to the line joining the first and fifth metatarsal heads.

Painful heels

Pain *under the heel*, for example from plantar fasciitis, may be relieved by fitting a horse-shoe shaped sponge rubber heel pad inside the shoe on a leather insole (Fig. 11.8). If the insole is not effective, it is possible to excavate the heel of a welted shoe and then to fill the cavity with sorbo rubber.

Pain over the *back of the heel* from an exostosis of the calcaneus can be relieved by removing the stiffener from the back of the shoe

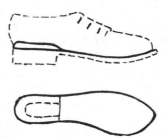

Figure 11.8 Heel pad. Note the horse-shoe shape to the sponge rubber pad.

and inserting two small thick sponge rubber pads covered with chamois leather, one on each side of the exostosis.

Painful toes

Deformed toes may give rise to pain due to pressure upon them by the shoe. This pressure may be relieved by stretching the shoe over the toes, but it may be necessary to prescribe surgical footwear to accommodate the deformities.

Hallux rigidus. The pain from hallux rigidus may be relieved by modifying the footwear so that dorsiflexion at the metatarsophalangeal joint of the hallux is reduced or eliminated. This can be achieved in two ways.

(1) *Rocker bar.* A rocker bar (Fig. 11.9) is added to the sole of the shoe or boot. Its apex lies just behind and parallel to the line joining the first and fifth metatarsal heads. It differs from a metatarsal bar in that its anterior extension is longer, its overall length being up to 2½ inches (5·6 cm).

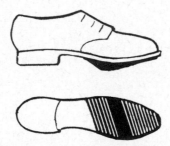

Figure 11.9 Rocker bar for hallux rigidus. Note that the apex of the bar lies immediately behind and parallel to the line joining the first and fifth metatarsal heads, *but that its anterior extension is longer than that of a metatarsal bar*. (Fig. 11.7).

(2) *Stiffening the medial side of the sole of the shoe.* In a shoe of welted construction, this can be achieved by inserting a steel plate (shank) 1 inch (2·5 cm) wide between the layers of the sole. The steel shank must extend well back into the waist of the shoe.

An alternative method, in a shoe of non-welted construction, is to add an extra layer of leather (not microcellular rubber) to the sole of the shoe. The additional stiffness these procedures confer, prevents dorsiflexion at the metatarso-phalangeal joint of the hallux.

Outside heel float

The lateral ligament of the ankle may be partially or completely ruptured following a severe inversion injury. This may result in the ankle being unstable and repeatedly suffering further inversion injuries.

In the absence of radiological evidence of increased talar tilt either with or without general anaesthesia, or if the patient should decline operative repair of the ligament, inversion injuries can be prevented by floating out the lateral side of the heel of the shoe (Fig. 11.10).

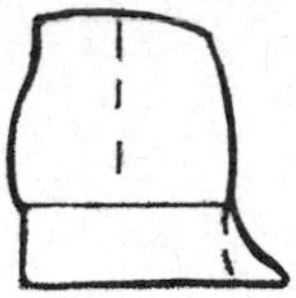

Figure 11.10 Outside heel float. In addition an outside heel wedge can be added when weakness of the peroneal muscles is present.

Normally the first part of the heel of the shoe to strike the ground is situated about one-quarter to one-half inch (0·6 to 1·25 cm) to the lateral side of the centre of the heel. By floating out the lateral side of the heel, the part of the heel which first strikes the ground is brought medially towards the mid-point of the now widened heel. This discourages the tendency to varus movement at the ankle and subtalar joints.

In muscle imbalance, when the peroneal muscles are weak, an outside heel float with possibly the addition of an outside heel wedge, or an inside below knee iron with an outside T strap, can be used to correct the varus deformity which occurs.

Toe blocks

Occasionally for multiple deformities, gangrene or infection, all the toes have to be amputated. Following this procedure a toe block is prescribed. It is made of sorbo rubber or Plastazote. In addition, a light steel or high density polyethylene (Ortholene) shank extending from the heel to the toe of the shoe must be fitted, to prevent the tip of the shoe from curling upwards.

TRUE AND APPARENT DISCREPANCY IN LENGTH OF THE LOWER LIMBS

In clinical practice, the exact length of each lower limb is relatively unimportant. What is important is the difference in length which may exist between the two limbs. This difference in length may be true or apparent, or a combination of both.

True discrepancy in length

True shortening of one lower limb is present when there is a decrease in the distance between the upper surface of the head of the femur and the lower surface of the calcaneus, compared with the other limb. This distance cannot be measured accurately by clinical means because of the deeply placed positions of the relevant bony points. Accurate measurement is possible only by taking a special radiograph—a scanograph—on which both lower limbs from the hips to the feet are shown alongside a scale.

For clinical purposes, the fixed bony points between which measurements are taken are the anterior superior iliac spine and the tip of the medial malleolus. It is accepted that the anterior superior iliac spine lies at a level proximal and lateral to the upper surface of the head of the femur, and that a part of the talus and calcaneus lies distal to the tip of the medial malleolus. This means that destruction of the superior lip of the acetabulum, or upward sub-luxation or dislocation of the head of the femur, will show as true shortening when in fact the distances between the upper surface of the head of the femur and the under surface of the calcaneus of both limbs are identical. In addition loss of limb length from a compression fracture of the calcaneus will not be identified.

Apparent discrepancy in length

Apparent discrepancy in length of the lower limbs is due to the presence of a fixed adduction or abduction deformity at one hip.

In normal walking or standing, the lower limbs are parallel. To bring the lower limbs into a parallel position when a fixed ad-duction or abduction deformity is present at one hip, the pelvis is tilted in one direction or the other (Fig. 11.11). In the presence of a fixed adduction deformity, the anterior superior iliac spine on the same side is raised above the horizontal, causing apparent shortening of the ipsilateral limb. When a fixed abduction deformity is present, the anterior superior iliac spine on the opposite side is raised above the horizontal, causing apparent shortening of the contralateral limb (or apparent lengthening of the ipsilateral limb).

The accurate measurement of apparent discrepancy in the length of the lower limb is unimportant clinically. What is important is that the detection of an apparent discrepancy in length indicates the presence of a fixed deformity at one hip.

MEASUREMENT OF THE TRUE LENGTH OF
THE LOWER LIMBS
With the patient supine
● Stand on the right-hand side of the patient.
● Identify both anterior superior iliac spines and draw an imaginary line joining these two points.
● Project a second line distally from the centre and at right angles to the line joining the anterior superior iliac spines.

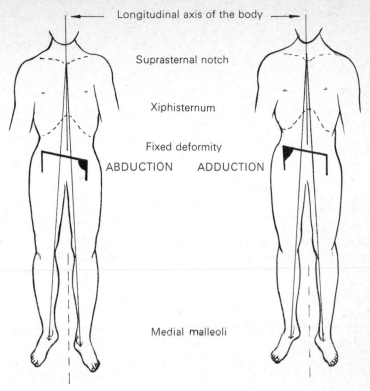

Longitudinal axis of the body

Suprasternal notch

Xiphisternum

Fixed deformity
ABDUCTION   ADDUCTION

Medial malleoli

Figure 11.11   Apparent discrepancy in length of one lower limb may be due to a fixed abduction or adduction deformity being present at one or the other hip joint.

The anterior superior iliac spine lies proximal and lateral to the upper surface of the head of the femur. This is of no significance if the long axis of each limb subtends the same angle with the line joining both anterior superior iliac spines. If, however, the angle is different on each side, the measurements will be misleading. Abduction of a limb approximates the anterior superior iliac spine and the medial malleolus, whereas adduction increases the distance between these two points (Fig. 11.12).

● Prior to measuring the true lengths, place the normal limb in a similar position to that of the affected limb. When a fixed adduction deformity is present at one hip, the affected limb will lie across the distally projected line (Fig. 11.13), and when a fixed abduction deformity is present, the affected limb will lie some distance away from this line (Fig. 11.14).

● Grip one end of a tape measure between the tips of the *left* index finger and thumb, so that the thumb nail is at right angles to the upper surface of the tape measure.

● Slip the left thumb and tape measure in an upward direction until the pulp of the thumb, covered by the end of the tape measure, impinges upon the lower surface of the anterior superior iliac spine.

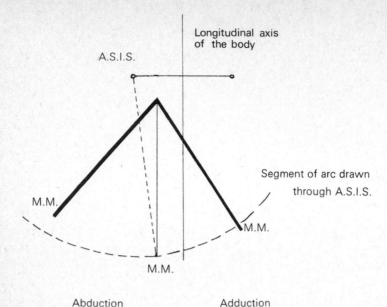

Figure 11.12 A.S.I.S. Anterior superior iliac spine; M.M. Medial malleolus. Abduction of the hip approximates the medial malleolus and the A.S.I.S., whereas adduction increases the distance between the medial malleolus and the A.S.I.S.

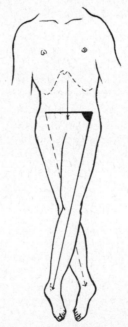

Figure 11.13 The position in which the lower limbs must be placed when measuring for *true length* in the presence of a fixed *adduction deformity* at one (here the left) hip.

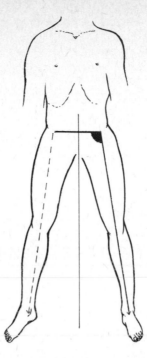

Figure 11.14   The position in which the lower limbs must be placed when measuring for *true length* in the presence of a fixed *abduction deformity* at one (here the left) hip.

Identify the anterior superior iliac spine in this manner, as the presence of overlying mobile subcutaneous fatty tissue will make the accurate identification of the anterior superior iliac spine impossible by any other means.

● Maintain the left thumb in contact with the anterior superior iliac spine and lay the tape measure evenly along the medial border of the patella, and then slide the *right* thumb down the tape measure until it slips over the lower margin of the medial malleolus.

● Note the reading on the tape measure.

● Maintain the same grip on the tape measure with the left hand, and repeat the manoeuvre for the opposite limb.

● Any difference between the two measurements indicates the amount of true shortening present.

With the patient standing

● Stand the patient erect with both knees fully extended.

● Identify both anterior superior iliac spines. The anterior superior iliac spine on the side of the shorter limb will lie at a lower level.

● Place wooden blocks of varying thickness under the foot of the shorter limb until the anterior superior iliac spines lie on a horizontal plane.

● The total height of the wooden blocks used equals the difference in limb length.

MEASUREMENT OF THE APPARENT LENGTH OF
THE LOWER LIMBS

The apparent lengths of the lower limbs are measured from a fixed
median point, such as the xiphisternum or suprasternal notch, to the
tips of the medial malleoli.

● Lay the patient supine.
● Ignoring the position of the pelvis, arrange the lower limbs evenly about
the longitudinal axis of the trunk, with only 3 to 4 inches (7·5 to
10 cm) between the medial malleoli (Fig. 11.11).
● Measure the distance from the xiphisternum or suprasternal notch to
the lower margin of each malleolus, handling the tape measure as
described above.
● A difference between the measurements for each lower limb indicates
the presence of a fixed adduction or abduction deformity at one hip,
but only if true shortening or lengthening is absent.

Compensation for a short lower limb

A short leg gait can be ungainly and tiring. In addition it can
increase the stresses imposed upon the hip joints and lumbo-sacral
spine and therefore contribute to the occurrence of pain at these
sites. Compensation for inequality in length of the lower limbs,
whether true or apparent, can improve function.

Before determining the height of raise required to compensate
for shortening of a lower limb, a number of facts must be taken
into consideration.

1. Does the patient have a fixed lateral curvature of the spine, or
   fixed pelvic obliquity? The presence of either of these deformities
   will influence the degree of pelvic tilt which can occur.
2. What is the range of flexion present at each hip? When one hip is
   arthrodesed, the patient can bring that limb forward during walking only by swinging the pelvis forward on the opposite hip. Unless
   sufficient clearance is allowed between the foot on the affected side
   and the ground, this will be impossible. Any raise supplied must
   be such that the affected limb is effectively one-half inch (1·25 cm)
   shorter than the other limb to give sufficient clearance.
3. What is the range of flexion present at each knee? Again any
   raise supplied must allow sufficient clearance—half an inch
   (1·25 cm)—to bring the affected limb forward.
4. What degree of fixed equinus (plantar flexion) of the ankle or
   forefoot is present? The degree of these deformities will determine
   the heights of the raises under the heel, the tread (metatarsal
   heads) and the toes.
5. What degree of mobility exists at the ankle and in the forefoot?
   As much equinus of the ankle and forefoot (pitch) as possible is
   allowed. This improves the appearance and decreases the weight
   of the footwear.

6. Is dorsiflexion at the metatarso-phalangeal joint of the hallux limited? Limitation of movement at this joint influences the amount of equinus of the ankle and forefoot which can be allowed. If too great a degree of equinus is allowed, the metatarso-phalangeal joint of the hallux will be forced into dorsiflexion. This may give rise to pain.

CALCULATION OF THE AMOUNT OF RAISE REQUIRED

It is rarely necessary to compensate for the first half an inch (1·25 cm) of shortening, as this amount can be accommodated easily by tilting the pelvis.

Although the theoretical height of the heel raise required to compensate for any shortening can be calculated by subtracting half an inch (1·25 cm) from the difference in length of the lower limbs measured with the patient supine, this method is unlikely to be satisfactory. All patients who require compensation for shortening must be measured in the standing position. In this position the height of the heel raise, and the degree of allowable equinus of the ankle and forefoot necessary to compensate for any true or apparent shortening, *which is comfortable to the patient*, can be determined. The comfort of the patient is much more important than any theoretical calculation.

● Stand the patient erect with both knees fully extended.
● Insert wooden blocks under the foot of the shorter limb. Blocks equal to the theoretical height of the required raise can be used initially.
● Tell the patient to mark time.
● Vary the thickness of the wooden blocks under the heel and tread until the patient is comfortable. Remind the patient to mark time between each variation in thickness of the wooden blocks.
● The ultimate thickness of the wooden blocks under the heel and tread equals the height of the raise required at these sites.

Note: The height of the heel raise is measured anterior to the *centre* of the heel of the shoe, that is, in line with the medial malleolus (Fig. 11.15). This means that when a raise is added to the heel of

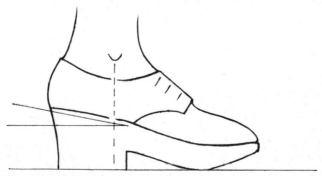

Figure 11.15   The height of a heel raise is measured in front of the centre of the heel, in line with the medial malleolus. Note that the heel raise must be higher posteriorly than anteriorly.

a shoe, the thickness of the posterior border of the heel must be greater than that of the anterior border, otherwise the under surface of the sole and heel will not make simultaneous contact with the ground when standing, and all the stress will be taken by the anterior border of the heel.

As it is necessary to provide a rocker action for walking, the height of the raise must decrease towards the toe (Fig. 11.16). The height of the raise at the toe will depend upon that at the tread. If this is large, the tapering must be more.

Occasionally after giving a patient a raise determined in the above way, the gait pattern may still be poor. Do not over-compensate for shortening to try to improve a gait pattern in the presence of adequate compensation for shortening, as the poor gait pattern may be due to weakness of the spinal or abdominal muscles.

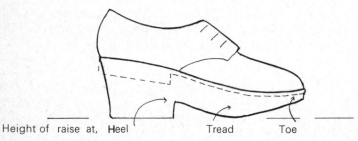

Height of raise at,   Heel   Tread   Toe

Figure 11.16   Outside raise. Note that the raise tapers towards the toe to aid walking.

TYPES OF RAISES EMPLOYED

Outside raise

If the foot is normal, the raise can be added to ordinary footwear. Sensible footwear is essential. Certain types of footwear are unsuitable for the addition of a raise, for example:

Shoes with heels exceeding 2 inches (5·0 cm) in height.

Court shoes. The addition of a raise to a court shoe causes loss of flexibility of the shoes with the result that the patient's heel tends to come out of the shoe.

Shoes with welded rubber soles and heels, as it is difficult to remove the original sole.

Veltshorn shoes are not suitable for a raise in excess of 1½ inches (3·75 cm).

When the required raise is one-quarter to three-quarters of an inch (0·6 to 2·0 cm), the heel and if necessary the sole can be raised by adding to the surface of the existing heel and sole. Microcellular rubber is used for the raise in preference to leather, as it is lighter, more flexible and wears better.

When a heel raise of more than three-quarters of an inch (2·0 cm) is required, the existing sole and heel are removed and layers of cork are added to obtain the required height. The cork layers are shaped and covered with leather similar to that of the shoe. The original sole and heel are reattached if possible, or if not, a new sole and heel are made (Figs. 11.16 and 11.17).

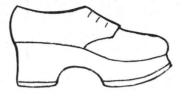

Figure 11.17   Outside raise—arched.

Inside raise

When a foot is deformed or of an odd size, surgical footwear must be made. In these cases, all or part of the raise may be concealed within the upper. This is known as an inside raise (Fig. 11.18). The maximum height for an inside raise is usually $3\frac{1}{2}$ inches (8·0 cm) at the heel, with 2 inches (5·0 cm) at the tread, and approximately 1 inch (2·5 cm) at the toe. If a larger raise than this is required, the additional height is obtained by adding an outside raise.

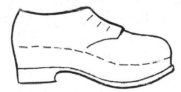

Figure 11.18   Inside raise in a surgical shoe.

When the required raise is more than $3\frac{1}{2}$ inches (8·0 cm), the cork raise can be arched and bridge waisted. The bridge, which must be strong and perhaps reinforced with a steel plate, prevents the heel and tread raises from splaying out on walking (Fig. 11.19).

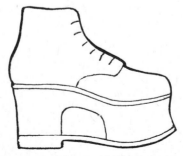

Figure 11.19   Outside raise arched and bridge waisted.

As has already been mentioned, as much equinus of the ankle and forefoot as possible is allowed. However, in such a situation the heel platform must be flat to prevent the patient's foot from sliding down the slope and the patient's toes impinging against the tip of the shoe.

REFERENCES

Tuck, W. H. (1971) Personal communication.

12. Walking aids

Walking aids are used to increase the mobility of a patient, as they enable some of the body weight to be supported by the upper limbs. There are many different walking aids—parallel bars, walking frames, crutches and sticks—and many different types within each broad group. The correct selection of a walking aid for a particular patient is very important and depends upon:

1. Stability of the patient.
2. Strength of the patient's upper and lower limbs.
3. Degree of co-ordination of movement of the upper and lower limbs.
4. Degree of relief from weight-bearing required.

These aids may be sufficient in themselves or they may have to be used in conjunction with calipers or other orthopaedic appliances.

As the condition of the patient improves he may progress through the different types of walking aids. Whether or not the ultimate aim of walking unaided is achieved will depend upon the degree of any permanent residual disability.

After a prolonged illness, many patients are generally weak. This can be minimised by good nutrition and a well planned progressive course of exercises. When a walking aid is used, part of the body weight is taken by the muscles of the shoulder girdles and upper limbs. Attention may have to be paid to the strength of these muscles when planning the rehabilitation of the patient. The particular muscles used are:

1. Flexors of the fingers and thumb to hold the handgrips firmly.
2. Dorsiflexors of the wrist to stabilise the wrist in dorsiflexion, thereby obtaining the best functional position for powerful finger flexion.
3. Extensors of the elbow to stabilise the elbow in slight flexion when the body weight is taken through the upper limb.
4. Flexors of the shoulder to move the walking aid forward.
5. Depressors of the shoulder girdle to support the body weight.

To regain confidence in walking takes time. When walking is commenced it is therefore important to eliminate the fear of falling and to avoid too rapid progression.

PARALLEL BARS

Parallel bars are rigid and do not have to be moved by the patient. This enables the patient to concentrate entirely on moving his lower limbs correctly. For this reason parallel bars are often used when the patient is not stable, or initially to develop a particular pattern of gait, the patient being taught the correct sequence of arm and lower limb movement.

A full-length mirror should be placed at one end of the parallel bars. In it the patient can observe his movements and thus avoid looking at his feet, a common mistake made when any type of walking aid is used initially. A mirror is particularly helpful if the patient has lost proprioception.

Adjustment: Some parallel bars are not adjustable. If they are, adjust the distance between the bars and the height of the bars so that when they are held by the patient his elbows are in 30 degrees of flexion.

WALKING-FRAMES

A patient is not usually given a walking-frame unless he will never be able to walk with walking-sticks, tripods or crutches, as the pattern of gait acquired in a walking-frame is difficult to change. Moreover, a patient who uses a walking-frame is usually confined to his home, and is unable to manage stairs. If parallel bars are not available, however, a walking-frame is very useful initially when a patient is unstable and fearful of falling.

There are three main types of walking-frame: the standard walking-frame, the reciprocal walking-frame and the rollator. The first two are usually used for elderly patients who lack confidence in walking and are unsteady. Walking with full or partial weight bearing is possible. The rollator is usually reserved for patients suffering from a neurological conditions, such as disseminated sclerosis, with incoordination of the lower limbs.

Standard walking-frame

The standard walking-frame (Fig. 12.1) is light, rigid, stable and easy to use. It consists of four almost vertical aluminium alloy tubes arranged in a rectangle, and joined together on three sides by upper and lower horizontal tubes. One long side of the rectangle is left open. The lower ends of the vertical tubes, which may be adjustable by means of spring-loaded double ball catches, are fitted with rubber tips. Hand-grips are fitted to the short, upper, horizontal tubes on each side.

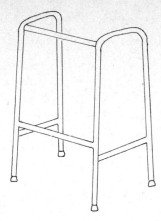

Figure 12.1   Walking frame.

Adjustment: If the frame is adjustable, alter the height of *all* the vertical tubes, and ensure that they are all of equal length, so that when the handgrips are held by the patient, the patient's elbows are in 30 degrees of flexion. Patients with incoordination of the lower limbs may find walking easier if the handgrips are higher.

How to use : The patient stands in the walking-frame, lifts and places the frame forward a short distance and then walks into the frame still holding the handgrips.

Reciprocal walking-frame

A reciprocal walking-frame is basically identical with a standard frame, except that each side of the frame can be moved forward alternately. There are swivel joints between the front horizontal and vertical tubes. As the frame does not have to be lifted clear of the ground with each step, the patient's stability is increased.

Adjustment: Adjust as for the standard walking-frame.

How to use : A four-point gait is used (see Chapter 13). One side of the frame is lifted and moved forward, the two legs of the other side remaining in contact with the ground.

Rollator

A rollator (Fig. 12.2) has two small wheels at the front and two short legs at the back, protected by rubber tips. The rear legs are almost vertically under the handgrips. Care must be taken when recommending a rollator for elderly patients as it may roll too far forward so that they lose their balance.

Adjustment: Adjust as for the standard walking-frame.

How to use : The patient holds the handgrips, lifts them to raise

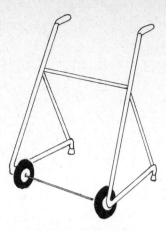

Figure 12.2   Rollator.

the rear legs just off the ground, wheels the rollator forward a short distance, lowers the rear legs onto the ground and then walks forward into the rollator still holding the handgrips.

CRUTCHES

There are three main types of crutches, axillary or underarm crutches, elbow crutches and gutter crutches.

Axillary crutches

The common axillary crutches (Fig. 12.3) are made of wood. They consist of a double upright joined at the top by a padded axillary portion, a handgrip, and a non-slip rubber tip covering the lower end. The overall length of the crutch and the position of the hand-grip should be adjustable. By using adjustable crutches, it is easier to fit each individual patient correctly, and the possible waste of cutting nonadjustable crutches to the correct size, is avoided.

When triceps weakness is present, support can be provided by attaching to the outer side of the crutch, above the level of the handgrip, a half-loop band between the double upright through which the upper arm is placed, or a short metal gutter piece to the posterior upright against which the upper arm is pressed backwards.

All degrees of weight relief are possible with axillary crutches. Usually they are used when crutch walking is commenced initially and when non-weight bearing on one lower limb is indicated, for example after a fracture. Although more cumbersome than elbow crutches, they are more stable. The patient can release a handgrip and use that hand to open a door or adjust his clothing, while continuing to support himself. This is important when the patient's balance is poor.

Methods of initial measurement of length for axillary crutches

It is necessary to be able to obtain some initial indication of the overall length of the crutches required by a particular patient. This measurement should be as accurate as possible. Final adjustment of the crutches for overall length and position of the handgrip, however, must be carried out with the patient standing and wearing shoes.

There are many methods of obtaining such a measurement. Beckwith (1965) states that the following two methods of measuring patients for axillary crutches are the most accurate.

1. Subtract 16 inches (41·0 cm) from the height of the patient, or
2. With the patient lying supine, measure the distance from the anterior axillary fold to the bottom edge of the heel of the shoe.

The measurement obtained with these two methods equals the overall length of the crutch from the top of the axillary pad to the bottom of the rubber tip.

ADJUSTMENT OF AXILLARY CRUTCHES

The overall length and the position of the handgrip must be correct for each patient.

When walking with crutches, patients wear shoes and the height of the heel will vary from patient to patient. With the patient standing up straight, the axillary crutches extend from a point 2 inches (5·0 cm) or three finger breadths below the anterior axillary fold, to a point on the ground 6 inches (15·0 cm) in front of and lateral to the tips of the toes. The shoulders are depressed and the palms of the hands rest on top of the handgrips with the elbows in 30 degrees of flexion. (See Crutch stance, Chapter 13.)

Adjustment must be carried out with the patient standing and wearing shoes.

● Place a crutch under each arm.
● Check that the palms of the hands are on top of the handgrips.
● Place the tips of the crutches on the ground 6 inches (15·0 cm) in front of and lateral to the tips of the toes.
● Ask the patient to stand up straight and to relax his shoulders.

Checking overall length

● Attempt to insert three fingers between the axillary pad and the anterior axillary fold.

Too long—Less than three fingers can be inserted between the axillary pad and the anterior axillary fold. The crutches are forced into the axilla, the shoulders are hunched and the patient is unable to lift his body off the ground. Pressure on the nerves in the axilla may cause paralysis.

Too short—More than three fingers can be inserted between the axillary pad and the anterior axillary fold. The patient leans forward from the waist, his buttocks project backwards and the line of his centre of gravity passes down in front of his feet. This position is potentially unstable. It could be corrected and the pelvis brought forward by maintaining some degree of hip and knee flexion. This must not be done as it is tiring and may hinder crutch walking.

To adjust the length of the crutch
- Take off the bottom two wing nuts and remove the bolts.
- Slide the crutch extension to the correct length.
- Replace the bolts and wing nuts, but do not tighten the wing nuts at this stage, otherwise it will be impossible to move the handgrip.
- Check the overall length of the crutch again.

Checking the position of the handgrip
With the shoulder depressed and the palm of the hand on top of the handgrip, the elbow should be in 30 degrees of flexion.

Too high—The elbows are flexed more than 30 degrees, the shoulders are hunched and the ability to grip the axillary pad between the upper arm and the side wall of the chest is lost.

Too low—The palms of the hands do not rest on top of the handgrips, the axillary pad presses into the axilla, the elbows are flexed less than 30 degrees and the ability to take weight on the hands is lost.

To adjust the position of the handgrip
- Remove the uppermost wing nut and bolt.
- Move the handgrip to the correct position.
- Replace the bolt and wing nut.
- Check that the elbow is in 30 degrees of flexion.
- *Tighten all the wing nuts.*

  Note : The axillary pad must be gripped between the upper arm and the side wall of the chest. The patient must not lean on the axillary pad otherwise paralysis may occur from pressure of the axillary pad on the nerves in the axilla.

Elbow crutches (Loftstrand crutches)

Most elbow crutches are made from a single adjustable tube of aluminium alloy to which are attached a U-shaped metal cuff (armband), to accommodate the forearm just below the elbow, and a rubber or plastic covered handgrip. The lower end is protected by a rubber tip (Fig. 12.3).

The armband is made usually from spring steel. It grips the forearm, thus enabling the crutch to be controlled when freedom of hand movement is required. The armband may have a front or side opening and may be fixed rigidly or be attached by a hinge joint

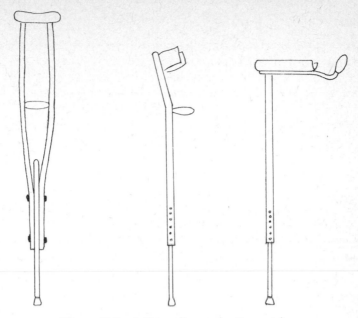

Figure 12.3   Axillary, elbow and gutter crutches.

to the upper end of the crutch. Armbands which are not made from spring steel and are rigidly fixed to the upper end of the crutch can be obtained also. Occasionally for young children the armband is replaced by a padded ring.

Adjustment of the length of the crutch between the lower end and the handgrip is by means of a spring-loaded double-ball catch, and this mechanism is also used in some crutches to vary the distance between the handgrip and the armband.

Heavy duty elbow crutches, made from stainless steel tubing, are available.

Elbow crutches are less cumbersome, and confer less stability than axillary crutches, but are more stable than walking-sticks. They are prescribed for patients who can take some weight on both feet but require an aid for balance and confidence, for example when partial weight bearing with the three-point crutch gait, the four-point crutch gait or the two-point crutch gait (see Chapter 13). Some patients with paraplegia, who have unusual skill, strength, co-ordination and balance, may be able to use elbow crutches with the swing-through gait.

ADJUSTMENT OF ELBOW CRUTCHES
Elbow crutches must be accurately adjusted for each patient. Adjustment must be carried out with the patient standing and wearing shoes.

When elbow crutches are adjusted correctly the tips of the crutches are on the ground 6 inches (15·0 cm) in front of and lateral to the tips of the toes and the patient is standing up straight, with his shoulders depressed and his elbows in 30 degrees of flexion.

● Ask the patient to put his arms through the armbands and to grasp the handgrips.
● Check that the palms of the hands are on top of the handgrips.
● Place the tips of the crutches on the ground, 6 inches (15·0 cm) in front of and lateral to the tips of the toes.
● Ask the patient to stand up straight and to relax his shoulders.

Checking overall length

Too long—The shoulder is hunched and the elbow is flexed more than 30 degrees.

Too short—The patient is leaning forwards and the elbow is flexed less than 30 degrees.

To adjust the length of the crutch

● Disengage the spring-loaded double-ball catch by pressing in both buttons.
● Slightly twist the lower part of the crutch so that about half of each button is visible.
● Slide the lower part of the crutch to the desired position.
● Twist back the lower part of the crutch to allow both buttons of the ball catch to jump out.
● Check that the lower part of the crutch is firmly locked in the new position.
● Check the overall length of the crutch again.

Checking the position of the armband

The position of the armband is correct when the gap between the top of the armband and the flexor crease of the elbow is 2 inches (5·0 cm).

Adjust the position of the armband if this is possible.

Gutter crutches

A gutter crutch (Fig. 12.3) consists of a single adjustable tube of aluminium alloy. Attached to the upper end is a short horizontal metal gutter or trough in which the forearm rests with the elbow in 90 degrees of flexion. Projecting forward from the gutter is an adjustable bar carrying a vertical handgrip. The gutter, which may be padded, is secured to the forearm by Velcro fastenings. On some crutches the angle between the gutter and the alloy tube and the position of rotation of the handgrip in relation to the gutter, may be adjusted. The lower end of the crutch is protected by a rubber tip. Adjustment of length is by means of a spring-loaded double-ball catch.

Gutter crutches are indicated when there is a fixed flexion

deformity of the elbow joint, weakness of the muscles controlling the elbow joint or hand, a deformity of the hand causing difficulty in gripping, or when the patient experiences pain in the hand or wrist on taking weight through the upper limb.

ADJUSTMENT OF GUTTER CRUTCHES
- Strap the forearm into the gutter so that the point of the elbow lies at or just behind the posterior edge of the gutter.
- Adjust the distance between the front of the gutter and the handgrip, so that the handgrip can be grasped firmly. If rotatory adjustment of the handgrip in relation to the gutter is possible, adjust.
- Ask the patient to stand up as straight as possible.
- Place the tip of the crutch on the ground 6 inches (15·0 cm) in front of and lateral to the tips of the toes.
- Adjust the height of the crutch by means of the spring-loaded double-ball catch so that the elbow is in 90 degrees of flexion. If the patient is unable to flex his elbow to 90 degrees, then a crutch in which the angle between the gutter and the crutch can be adjusted is required.

WALKING-STICKS

The commonly used walking-stick is made of wood, with a C-curved handle; a right-angled or pistol-grip handle is also available and may be preferred by the patient. A rubber tip protects the lower end. Adjustable sticks made from aluminium alloy tubing with rubber or moulded plastic handgrips can be obtained.

Walking-sticks are not as stable as elbow crutches, but are lighter and more easily stored. They assist balance and provide moderate support for a lower limb, and thus can improve gait and help to relieve pain, for example from a painful hip. Walking-sticks are not used unless the disabled lower limb can bear weight.

Choosing the correct walking-stick
A patient when using a walking-stick should have his elbow in 30 degrees of flexion.

Too long—The shoulder is elevated, the elbow is flexed more than 30 degrees, ulnar deviation of the wrist is increased unless the grip on the handle is changed and support is decreased.

Too short—The patient leans forward and the elbow is flexed less than 30 degrees.

ADJUSTMENT OF WALKING-STICKS
- Place the handle of the walking-stick on the ground beside the heel of the patient's shoe.
- Remove the rubber tip.

- Adjust the length of the walking-stick so that its (lower) end is level with the most prominent part of the greater trochanter or radial styloid process.
- Replace the rubber tip.
- Reverse the walking-stick and check that the patient's elbow is in 30 degrees of flexion.

TRIPOD AND QUADRUPED WALKING AIDS

These walking aids are similar. They are made from aluminium alloy or steel tubing.

The TRIPOD WALKING AID (Fig. 12.4) has three rubber-tipped legs which touch the ground at the corners of an equilateral triangle. The looped or right-angled handgrip lies in the same plane as a line joining two of the legs. The height of the handgrip can be adjusted.

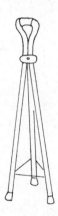

Figure 12.4 Tripod walking aid.

The QUADRUPED WALKING AID has four rubber-tipped legs. The handgrip lies vertically above the two inner legs, which are more widely spaced than the two outer legs. The height of the handgrip is adjustable.

The tripod and quadruped walking aids, which may be used singly or in pairs, confer more stability than walking-sticks or elbow crutches. They cannot pivot forwards and must be lifted and placed in a forward position. This requires more strength in the upper limbs than would be required for walking-sticks or crutches. Usually they are reserved for patients suffering from neurological conditions, but they may be used in the rehabilitation of elderly patients who have sustained injury to their lower limbs. These walking aids have one particular advantage over walking-sticks and crutches; they will stand upright beside a bed or a chair, ready for use.

ADJUSTMENT OF TRIPOD OR QUADRUPED WALKING AIDS

- Place the walking aid beside the patient, and ask him to take hold of the handgrip.
- Check that the aid is correctly orientated. *The handgrip must lie vertically above the two legs which are nearest to and parallel to the patient's foot* (Fig. 12.5). If the aid is positioned incorrectly, the patient will trip over the legs of the aid which lie, or will come to lie with use, in front of the patient's foot.

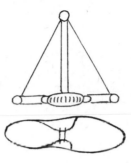

Figure 12.5   Correct orientation of tripod walking aid. Note that the handgrip must lie vertically above the two legs of the walking aid which are nearest to and parallel to the patient's foot.

- Check that the palm of the hand lies on top of the handgrip.
- Check that the handgrip is at the correct height.
  Too high—the patient's elbow is flexed more than 30 degrees.
  Too low—the patient's elbow is flexed less than 30 degrees.
  To adjust the height of the handgrip
- Loosen the adjusting screw or disengage the spring-loaded double-ball catch.
- Raise or lower the handgrip to the correct level.
- Tighten the adjusting screw or ensure that the two buttons of the ball catch are engaged.
- Check that the handgrip lies parallel to the line joining the two inner legs.
- Push down *yourself* on the handgrip to ensure that the aid will not collapse.
- Check again that the handgrip is at the correct height.

HANDGRIPS

The handgrips of all walking aids can be modified to accommodate a stiff or deformed hand. The girth of a handgrip can be increased by wrapping lengths of orthopaedic felt or sponge rubber around it.

For a deformed hand, such as may occur in rheumatoid arthritis, a mould of the grip of that hand can be taken in Plastazote* and later be transferred to the handgrip of the appliance.

RUBBER TIPS

The suction-type tip is best (Fig. 12.6). It is flexible and the sides of the tip flare out slightly. There are concentric rubber rings on

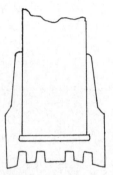

Figure 12.6   Cross-section of a rubber suction tip.

the undersurface, with the outermost ring projecting slightly beyond the other rings. On a wet surface these concentric rings exert a suction-cup effect. The flexibility of the tip and the suction-cup effect ensure that the undersurface of the tip comes into uniform contact with the ground even when the walking-stick or crutch is inclined at a slight angle from the vertical.

Hard small rubber tips, or worn suction tips are dangerous. They are likely to slip. They must be replaced.

REFERENCES

BECKWITH, J. M. (1965) Analysis of methods of teaching axillary crutch measurement. *Journal of the American Physical Therapy Association*, **45**, 1060.

* See Appendix.

13. Crutch walking

The majority of patients approach crutch walking with some apprehension, and the older and the more disabled the patient, the greater the apprehension. Sometimes crutches are needed only temporarily; at other times their need is permanent. The patient's ability to use crutches efficiently and perhaps eventually to walk unaided depends upon a number of factors.

1. The strength of the muscles required in the use of crutches (see Chapter 12).
2. The correct selection and adjustment of the crutches (see Chapter 12).
3. A good sense of balance.
4. Familiarity with the crutches and their maintenance.
5. The correct crutch stance.
6. Instruction in how to stand and balance with crutches before taking any steps.
7. The pattern of gait employed.
8. The initial development of the gait pattern between parallel bars if necessary.
9. Instruction and practice in walking and the performance of various manoeuvres essential for daily living, with the crutches.

CRUTCH MAINTENANCE

1. The wood or metal must not be cracked.
2. All the adjusting nuts must be tight, and all the spring-loaded double-ball catches must be working.
3. The rubber tips must be in good condition. If the tip is badly worn it must be replaced.
4. The handgrips and axillary pads if present, must be in good condition.

CRUTCH STANCE—AXILLARY CRUTCHES

Before taking any steps with the crutches, the patient must be instructed in how to stand and balance with them. This is achieved by standing the patient against a wall and placing a crutch under each arm. The correct stance with crutches is in a position with the head up, the back straight with the pelvis over the feet as much as possible, the shoulders depressed not hunched, the axillary pads of the crutches gripped between the upper arms and the side walls of the chest 2 inches (5·0 cm) below the anterior axillary fold, the crutch tips 6 inches (15·0 cm) forward and 6 inches (15·0 cm) out from the tips of the toes, the palms of the hands on top of the handgrips, the body weight taken mainly on the hands, and the elbows in a position of 30 degrees of flexion.

The correct crutch stance with elbow or gutter crutches is basically the same.

CRUTCH WALKING—PATTERNS OF GAIT

There are four different patterns of gait.

1. Swinging crutch gaits.
2. Four-point crutch gait.
3. Two-point crutch gait.
4. Three-point crutch gait.

The patterns of gait employed with crutches differ in the combination of crutch and foot or crutches and feet movements used in taking steps, and in the sequence of such combinations.

To select the pattern of gait to be employed by a particular patient, the ability of the patient to step forward with either one or both feet, to bear weight and keep his balance on one or both lower limbs, to push his body off the ground by pressing down on both crutches, to maintain his body erect, and to control the crutches must be evaluated.

The pattern of gait which is selected should be as near normal as possible, consistent with the patient's condition. It is important to remember that walking aids are used to increase the patient's mobility. Each patient must be encouraged to walk even if he does not use a recognised pattern of gait. Any mobility is better than immobility.

It is impossible to teach any definite pattern of crutch walking to children under the age of five years. Children over the age of five can be taught but when they are alone they may not practise what they have been taught.

A distance of 12 inches (30·0 cm) is advocated as the length of step and of forward movement of the crutches when the sequence of movement in the different types of gait is described, in order to emphasise that these forward movements are small and equal. It is recognised that the length of step will vary with the height of the patient. It is important that any patient who is learning to use crutches should gain confidence as quickly as possible. Confidence will be gained more quickly if the initial steps are small. As confidence increases, the length of step can be increased. When the ground is wet or slippery, short steps are advisable as slipping will be less likely to occur.

Swinging crutch gaits

There are two types of swinging crutch gait, the swing-to crutch gait and the swing-through crutch gait. These gaits are used when the body weight can be taken through both lower limbs together but the patient is incapable of moving his lower limbs individually due to paralysis. Calipers are frequently worn to stabilise the lower limbs. The lower limbs are moved by the trunk muscles acting on the pelvis.

The stable position is that of a tripod, with a large triangular base and the apex at the shoulders. The two anterior legs of the tripod are formed by the backward and inward slanting crutches. The posterior leg of the tripod is formed by the trunk and lower limbs of the patient as he leans forward on the crutches. A patient, paralysed below the waist, is stable in this position provided that flexion contractures of the hip, knee, or ankle joints are not present, the knees are braced in extension and the centre of gravity falls in front of the hip joints, to maintain them passively in extension. If the centre of gravity falls behind the hip joints, passive hip extension will be lost, the hips will flex and the patient will collapse. Before attempting to progress the patient must practise standing in this position until he has acquired a sufficiently good sense of balance to give him confidence.

In the swing-to crutch gait, the patient advances the crutches and then swings his body to the crutches. In the swing-through crutch gait the body is swung through beyond the crutches.

Swing-to crutch gait
Crutch–foot sequence : Both crutches; lift and swing the body to the crutches.

The patient is in the stable position.

- Place both crutches forward together a short distance.
- Take all the body weight on the hands and at the same time straighten the elbows to lift the body.
- Swing both lower limbs forward together *to between the crutches*, arching the spine as the heels touch the ground first.

- Keep the spine arched and the hips well forward. This will maintain the hips and knees in extension and stabilise the lower limbs.
- Take the body weight on both feet.
- *Immediately* place both crutches forward a distance of 12 inches (30·0 cm) *in front of the feet*, to regain the stable position.
- Repeat the above.

Initially, patients may not have either the confidence or the power in the upper limbs or trunk to perform the swing-to crutch gait as described above. When this occurs, the patient is taught to hitch the crutches forward and then to slide, jerk or drag the feet forward together by a body movement, while bearing down on the hand-grips and keeping the body inclined forward sufficiently to maintain the centre of gravity in front of the hip joints. As confidence and strength improve, the swing-to crutch gait will develop.

Swing-through crutch gait

Crutch–foot sequence : Both crutches; lift and swing the body beyond the crutches.

The swing-through crutch gait, although quicker than the swing-to crutch gait, must be attempted only when the patient's balance is excellent.

The patient is in the stable position.

- Place both crutches forward together a short distance.
- Take all the body weight on the hands and at the same time straighten the elbows to lift the body.
- Swing both lower limbs forward together *through the crutches*, arching the spine as the heels touch the ground first, 12 inches (30·0 cm) *in front of the crutches*.
- Keep the spine arched and the hips well forward.
- Take the body weight on both feet. The forward momentum brings the trunk and the crutches to the erect position.
- *Immediately* place both crutches forward a distance of 12 inches (30·0 cm) *in front of the feet*, to regain the stable position.
- Repeat the above.

Four-point crutch gait

Crutch–foot sequence : Right crutch; left foot; left crutch; right foot.

The four-point crutch gait is used when all or part of the body weight can be taken on each foot, but the patient is unsteady and therefore requires a wide base of support. As the patient's balance improves, he may progress to the two-point crutch gait.

The patient is standing on BOTH feet with a crutch under each arm.

- Place the *left crutch* forward a distance of 12 inches (30·0 cm).
- Step forward 12 inches (30·0 cm) with the *right foot*, taking part of the body weight on the left hand.
- Place the *right crutch* forward a distance of 12 inches (30·0 cm) *in front of the left crutch*.
- Step forward with the *left foot*, placing it 12 inches (30·0 cm) *in front of the right foot*, taking part of the body weight on the right hand.
- Repeat the above.

Two-point crutch gait

Crutch–foot sequence : Right crutch and left foot simultaneously; left crutch and right foot simultaneously.

When the two-point crutch gait is used the amount of body weight taken on both feet is reduced. This type of gait is used when the patient's balance is good, some body weight can be taken through both lower limbs but both lower limbs are painful or weak.

The patient is standing on BOTH feet with a crutch under each arm.

- Place the *right crutch* and the *left foot* forward together a distance of 12 inches (30·0 cm), taking part of the body weight on the left foot.
- Place the *left crutch* and the *right foot* forward together a distance of 12 inches (30·0 cm) *in front of the left foot*, taking part of the body weight on the right foot.
- Repeat the above.

Three-point crutch gait

Crutch–foot sequence : Both crutches and the weaker lower limb together; the stronger lower limb.

By using the three-point crutch gait, the amount of body weight taken by a foot can vary from none to partial or full. The three-point crutch gait is commonly taught to orthopaedic patients who may have one painful or weak lower limb which cannot support the whole body weight, and one lower limb which can. Both crutches support the weaker lower limb, while the stronger lower limb takes the whole body weight without any support from the crutches.

The sequence of movement of the crutches and the lower limbs in performing different functions is described below.

Walking, non-weight bearing

The patient is standing on his RIGHT foot with a crutch under each arm : the LEFT foot is off the ground.

- Take all the body weight on the *right* foot.
- Place *both* crutches forward together a distance of 12 inches (30·0 cm).

- Carry the *left* lower limb forward to a position between the crutches with the left foot off the ground. As confidence increases both crutches and the left lower limb can be advanced together.
- Take the body weight on the hands and at the same time carry the pelvis forward to between the crutches. By this means the centre of gravity passes downwards through a line between the two crutches.
- Carry the *right* foot forward and place it on the ground 12 inches (30·0 cm) *in front of* the crutches. Do not fall forwards.
- Take all the body weight on the *right* foot.
- Repeat the above.

By carrying the pelvis forward to a position between the crutches before the right foot leaves the ground, a more stable position is obtained as the pendular movement of the pelvis and lower limb is reduced and excess forward swing is avoided.

When non-weight bearing in an above-knee plaster cast, it may be necessary to add a raise to the opposite shoe, especially if the knee is held extended, to ensure that the injured limb will clear the ground as it is brought forward. If a raise is not added, the injured limb will have to be carried in front of the body with the hip in slight flexion. To ensure non-weight bearing in young children it is essential to add a raise to the opposite shoe.

When a lower limb is strong enough to take part of the body weight, that limb is placed on the ground *at the same time as the two crutches*. By this means part of the body weight is taken on the hands, and part through the lower limb. This is termed partial weight bearing.

Getting up from a chair
Crutches; weak LEFT lower limb.

- Bring the heel of the *right* foot backwards to lie under the edge of the chair.
- Slide forwards on the chair so that the buttocks are resting on the edge of the chair.
- With the *right* hand, grip the arm of the chair as far forward as possible.
- Take hold of the handgrips of *both* crutches with the *left* hand.
- Place both crutches vertically on the floor near the front edge of the chair.
- Stand up by pushing upwards with the *right* leg and both arms, keeping the left foot off the ground.
- Transfer one crutch to the right hand.
- Place the crutches under the arms.
- Pause before walking to ensure that balance has been obtained.

When getting up from a wheelchair, check that the wheels are locked.

Sitting down in a chair
Crutches; weak LEFT lower limb.

- After reaching the chair, check that the chair is stable. This particularly applies to wheelchairs.
- Turn round so that the *back* of the *right* leg touches the front of the chair. This aids balance.
- Take the crutches from under the arms.
- Transfer the *right* crutch to the left hand.
- Hold *both* crutches in the *left* hand.
- Place the *right hand* on the arm of the chair.
- Bend forward slightly.
- Gently lower the body onto the chair.

Stepping up a kerb or step
The method described here is used also when going up stairs using two crutches.
Always step up with the stronger lower limb first.
Crutches; weak LEFT lower limb.

- Approach the kerb.
- Place the ends of *both* crutches in the angle formed by the kerb and the road.
- Take the body weight on the hands, straighten the elbows and carry the pelvis forward to between the crutches.
- Lift the *right* foot off the ground and carry it upwards and forwards onto the kerb.
- Straighten the right knee, thereby transferring the body weight on to the right foot.
- Lift *both* crutches up and carry them and the left lower limb forwards in preparation for the next step.

Stepping down a kerb or step
The following method is used also when going down stairs using two crutches.
Always step down with the crutches and the weaker lower limb together first.
Crutches; weak LEFT lower limb.

- Approach the edge of the kerb.
- Take all the body weight on the *right* foot.
- Place *both* crutches downwards and 12 inches (30·0 cm) forward on the road, bending the right knee and carrying the left lower limb forward at the same time. The higher the kerb, the greater the distance the crutches must be placed away from the kerb.
- Take the body weight on both hands and carry the pelvis forward to between the crutches.
- Lift the right foot off the ground and place it downwards and forwards on the road *in front of the crutches*, thus proceeding to the next step.

Ascending stairs with a handrail
Crutches; weak LEFT lower limb; handrail on the RIGHT.

- Approach the bottom of the stairs.
- Transfer the *right crutch* to the left hand. It is more convenient if the *transferred* crutch is carried horizontally in the left hand.
- Take a forward grip on the handrail with the *right* hand.
- Without moving the *left* crutch, lift the body upwards and forwards with both hands and at the same time lift the *right* foot upwards and forwards onto the first step.
- Lift the left crutch up on to the *same* step.
- Repeat the procedure until the top of the stairs is reached.
- Transfer the second crutch back under the right arm before proceeding.

If the handrail is on the left, the procedure is identical except that the left crutch is transferred to the right hand. Always step up with the stronger lower limb first.

Descending stairs with a handrail
Crutches; weak LEFT lower limb; handrail on the RIGHT.

- Approach the top of the stairs.
- Transfer the *right crutch* to the left hand, holding the transferred crutch horizontally.
- Place the *right* hand slightly forward on the handrail.
- Place the left crutch on the step below, bringing the left lower limb forward at the same time.
- Bend the *right knee* to bring the pelvis forward between the crutch and the right hand.
- Take the body weight on the hands.
- Lift the right foot off the ground and place it forwards and downwards on the same step as the left crutch.
- Repeat the procedure until the bottom of the stairs is reached.
- Transfer the second crutch back under the right arm before proceeding.

If the handrail is on the left, the procedure is identical except that the left crutch is transferred to the right hand. Always step down with the crutch and the weaker lower limb first.

Before a patient can be considered to be really efficient with crutches, he must be able to step backwards, forwards and sideways, and to walk on uneven surfaces and up and down inclines.

WALKING-STICKS

Walking-sticks can be used to decrease the amount of body weight taken through a lower limb during walking and therefore can compensate for muscle weakness and relieve pain. In addition the use of a walking-stick or sticks can increase the stability and the confidence of a patient.

Once a lower limb is strong enough to be able to take nearly all the body weight, two sticks can be substituted for crutches. The technique of walking with two sticks is the same as that described above for partial weight bearing with crutches. It is preferable to use two walking-sticks initially. If only one walking-stick is used, the patient will tend to lean towards the stick, to take a shorter stride on that side and to carry the opposite lower limb in abduction. This abnormal gait tends to persist after the walking-stick is abandoned. When a good technique using two walking-sticks has been achieved, one stick can be discarded. *The single walking-stick is carried in the opposite hand to the affected lower limb.* (Some patients, however, with a lesion of the knee or ankle, may gain more relief by holding the walking-stick in the ipsilateral hand.) For example, to obtain partial relief from weight bearing on the *left* foot, hold the walking-stick in the *right hand,* and place the left foot and the walking-stick forwards together at the same time.

Increased stability and further relief from weight bearing can be obtained by bringing the hand inward to rest against the body in the region of the greater trochanter of the femur.

14. Plaster-of-Paris casts

Plaster-of-Paris casts can be responsible for the development of serious complications.

IMPAIRMENT OF CIRCULATION

A limb which has been fractured, or upon which an operation has been performed, will always swell to a greater or lesser degree because of haemorrhage from the bone and surrounding traumatised soft tissue, and because of reactionary tissue oedema. If such a limb has been encased in a plaster cast the swelling can result in an appreciable increase in pressure within the cast, and cause a reduction in or the obliteration of the blood supply of the muscles and nerves. An increase in the pressure within a fascial compartment of the limb in the absence of a plaster cast can have the same result. This *impairment of the circulation can occur in the presense of distal peripheral pulses*. Ischaemia causes tissue death and subsequent fibrosis. Joint contracture, muscle paralysis and altered cutaneous sensibility may develop and cause considerable permanent impairment of the future function of that limb.

Patients who have sustained a fracture or undergone an operation commonly suffer pain. This pain rapidly and progressively decreases over the following two to three days. The persistence, the increase, or the recurrence of pain in an injured limb may herald the onset of circulatory impairment, or the development of a pressure sore.

Circulatory embarrassment or the development of a pressure sore is accompanied by severe pain. It is important to remember that patients do not always complain of pain to the attending doctor for varying reasons. Therefore, *every patient who has a plaster cast applied must be directly questioned as to the presence of pain. Do not wait for the patient to complain of pain—it may then be too late.*

TO PREVENT VASCULAR COMPLICATIONS
● Do not apply an unpadded plaster cast to a recently fractured limb. Many fractures can be adequately immobilised initially by the application over padding of a partly encircling plaster slab, the slab being retained by an encircling bandage. If a complete plaster cast must be used to maintain position, the plaster must be applied over padding. Preferably the plaster cast then should be split throughout its length.

● After an operation, always apply a well padded plaster cast, or split a lightly padded cast throughout its length.

● Elevate the encased limb so that gravity can assist the venous return from the limb.

● Encourage active finger and toe movements, again to assist the venous return.

● **Keep a frequent and careful check upon the state of the circulation in the affected limb.**

1. Enquire about the presence and site of any pain. *Never ignore the complaint of pain,* as even a fussy patient can develop circulatory embarrassment or a pressure sore.

2. Examine the fingers or toes for swelling. Swelling may be due to venous obstruction, dependancy of the injured limb, insufficient active exercise or a combination of all three.

3. Compare the state of the capillary circulation, especially in the nail beds, in the injured limb with that in the uninjured limb. Blanching on pressure should be followed by a quick return of colour on release of the pressure. The colour should be pink. Blueness of the extremities suggests venous obstruction. It should disappear on elevation of the limb. White and cold fingers or toes suggest arterial obstruction.

4. The peripheral pulses may be obscured by the cast, but where possible palpate them and compare with the uninjured limb. Remember that circulatory embarrassment can be present even when the distal pulses are palpable.

5. Examine the extremities for the presence of altered skin sensibility—hypoaesthesia.

6. Test the ease and range of active and passive movement of the fingers and toes. Pain on passive extension of the fingers or toes is strongly indicative of ischaemia of the flexor muscle groups.

If there is evidence of impairment of the circulation in a limb, the plaster cast must be split throughout its length, or removed completely at once. If impairment is due to a rise of pressure within a fascial compartment, then the limb must be decompressed immediately. Remember that the splitting or removal of a plaster cast may not be sufficient; the limb may also need to be decompressed. The delay of a few hours may have disastrous consequences. A good rule is if in doubt split the plaster cast: it is better to split a cast unnecessarily and possibly lose the position, than to run the risk of ischaemic changes occurring in a limb.

In general a lower limb cast is split along the front, and an upper limb cast along the ulnar or flexor surface. How to split a plaster cast is described later.

PRESSURE SORES

Pressure sores can develop under a plaster cast due to irregularity of the inner surface of the cast, insufficient padding especially over bony prominences, the presence of foreign bodies such as coins or matchsticks between the cast and the skin, or from the chafing of the skin by the rough edges of a crack in the cast. The development of pressure sores can be prevented by the careful application of adequate padding, by the avoidance of varying tension in a roll of padding or plaster as it is being applied, and by the avoidance of localised areas of pressure by fingers or thumb while the plaster is wet. With regard to the latter, a wet cast must be held only in the palm of the hand, so that pressure is spread over a wide area. In addition a wet cast must be supported throughout its length on a pillow until it is dry, to avoid direct pressure on an underlying bony prominence, such as the heel or the point of the elbow.

Diagnosis of the presence of a pressure sore

1. *Pain.* Pressure sores are painful initially. The pain will decrease when full thickness skin ulceration occurs. If a patient complains of pain under a plaster cast, which is not referable to the fracture or operation, the presence of a pressure sore must be suspected.
2. *Fretfulness* especially in children. Children may be too young to complain of localised pain.
3. *Disturbed sleep.* This again particularly applies to children.
4. *Rise in temperature.*
5. *Recurrence of swelling of the fingers and toes* once the initial swelling has subsided.
6. *The presence of an offensive smell*
7. *Discharge.* A discharge may present either from under the edge of the cast or by the appearance of a stain on a previously clean area of the cast.

By the time the patient exhibits a rise in temperature, or there is a recurrence of swelling of the fingers or toes, or an offensive smell or discharge is noted, full thickness skin ulceration with possibly necrosis of the underlying fat and muscle will have occurred. The presence of a pressure sore must be diagnosed before this state is reached.

If the presence of a pressure sore is suspected, the skin in that area must be examined immediately either by cutting a window, or by removing the cast altogether (these procedures are described in detail later). It is better to lose position rather than allow a pressure sore to develop.

INSTRUCTIONS TO AN OUT-PATIENT WEARING A PLASTER CAST

Only a small number of patients who have had a plaster cast applied are admitted to hospital. The vast majority are treated as out-patients.

Before any patient is allowed to leave hospital, the circulation in the encased limb must be checked and found to be satisfactory. In addition the patient must be given the following instructions both verbally and in writing.

1. The time and place of his next out-patient attendance which must be within the following twenty-four hours.
2. The patient must reattend immediately at any time of the day or night if he experiences severe pain or if his fingers or toes become blue, white or badly swollen.
3. The encased limb must be kept well elevated.
4. Active movements of his fingers or toes as well as all the joints not immobilised by the plaster cast must be carried out at regular frequent intervals.
5. Excessive local pressure on the plaster cast must be avoided.
6. The plaster cast must be kept dry.
7. The patient must reattend if the plaster cast shows evidence of cracking or softening.
8. If any object such as a coin or pencil is dropped under the cast, the patient must reattend immediately.

The application of the different plaster casts used in the treatment of fractures and other conditions is not described. This is well described in other books (*Plaster-of-Paris Technique: Gypsona Technique: Orthopaedic Nursing*).

The following procedures are described.

Removing a plaster cast.

Pre-operative preparation of a limb immobilised in a plaster cast.

Cutting a window in a plaster cast.

Splitting a plaster cast.

Wedging a plaster cast.

REMOVING A PLASTER CAST

A plaster cast used for the external immobilisation of a fracture will be removed after a certain number of weeks, to determine the state of union clinically and radiologically. When a plaster cast is removed, it is important that the skin of the limb is not damaged, the patient is not subjected to pain, and control of the fracture is maintained until it is decided that the cast can be discarded.

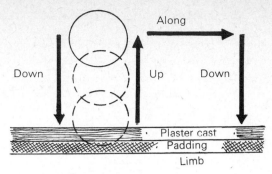

Figure 14.1   The correct way to use an electric plaster saw.

The plaster cast can be cut with plaster shears or with an electric plaster saw (e.g. Zimmer). Generally shears are used for children, small casts, and casts on the upper limbs. *The electric plaster saw must not be used on unpadded casts.* It may be used with great care when there is only stockinette under the cast.

HOW TO USE AN ELECTRIC PLASTER SAW (Fig. 14.1)

The cutting blade of an electric plaster saw does not rotate. It oscillates, and will damage the skin only if it is drawn along the limb or if the skin is adherent to the underlying bone and therefore not mobile.

- Switch on the saw.
- With light pressure apply the cutting blade to the plaster cast, keeping a finger under the neck of the saw to control the depth of the cut. In this way it is easy to feel when the saw has cut through the cast.
- Remove the blade from the cut formed in the cast.
- Reapply the cutting blade at a slightly higher or lower level.
- Repeat these separate and distinct movements until the cast has been divided along its length.

   Do not draw the cutting blade of an electric plaster saw along the limb, otherwise the skin will be cut. Take particular care when there is a blood-soaked dressing under the cast.

   Do not hold the electric saw with wet hands, or allow the lead to the saw to get wet.

HOW TO REMOVE A PLASTER CAST (Fig. 14.2)

- Determine if the cast is padded.
- Choose a line along which to cut the cast, avoiding any bony prominences, to reduce the risk of skin damage. For a lower limb cast, the line must pass in front of the lateral malleolus and behind the medial malleolus.
- Cut the cast on both sides of the limb (*bivalve*), with care.
- Remove the front half of the cast, divide the underlying padding, then carefully lift the limb out of the back half of the cast.
- Reapply the bivalved cast for transport to the Radiology Department.

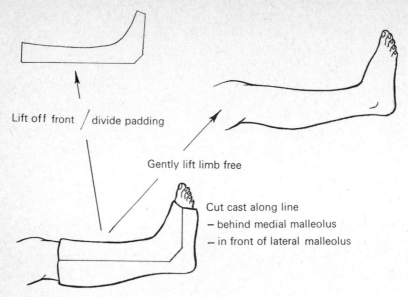

Lift off front / divide padding

Gently lift limb free

Cut cast along line
— behind medial malleolus
— in front of lateral malleolus

Figure 14.2 Bivalving a plaster cast.

PRE-OPERATIVE PREPARATION OF A LIMB IMMOBILISED IN A PLASTER CAST

It may be necessary to operate upon a limb which has been immobilised for some weeks in a plaster cast. Before operation, the skin should be prepared to remove the dead superficial epidermis and hair. After a few weeks a fractured limb can be moved painlessly with gentleness and care.

> PROCEDURE
> - Bivalve the cast as described above.
> - Gently remove the limb from the cast and place it on a sheet of polythene covered with a towel.
> - Gently wash the limb with soap and water, if necessary using a soft nail brush, to remove the scaly skin.
> - Shave the limb as necessary.
> - Wrap the limb in a sterile towel and replace it in the bivalved cast.
> - Apply a crepe bandage or lengths of zinc oxide strapping to hold the cast together.

CUTTING A WINDOW IN A PLASTER CAST

It is sometimes necessary to expose a limited area of skin surface for examination, when it is inadvisable to remove or bivalve the whole cast. This can be achieved by cutting a window in the cast.

When it is known that a window will be cut later in a cast, for example for the removal of sutures, the site of the window can be indicated by applying additional dressings or a pad of wool over the wound, so that an elevation in the cast is produced.

PROCEDURE (Fig. 14.3)
Removing the window
- Identify and mark out on the cast the area of skin to be exposed, allowing a reasonable margin for error.
- Cut along the marks with an electric plaster saw.
- Gently lever the window out.
- Remove the underlying padding to expose the skin.

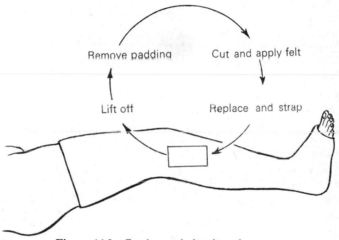

Figure 14.3   Cutting a window in a plaster cast.

Replacing the window
The window must be replaced after examination, otherwise, if the limb swells, the skin will impinge against the cut edges of the cast and pressure sores will result. In addition the cast will be weakened.
- Remove any padding from the undersurface of the window.
- Cut a piece of orthopaedic felt to the exact size of the window, and stick it onto the undersurface of the window.
- Replace the window.
- Firmly apply zinc oxide strapping or plaster bandage around the cast to retain the window in position.

SPLITTING A PLASTER CAST

HOW TO SPLIT A PLASTER CAST
- *Make a longitudinal cut through the cast from one end to the other*, using plaster shears or an electric plaster saw.
  Note that it is useless and dangerous to nibble at the free edge of the cast under the misunderstanding that the swelling of the fingers or toes

is due to constriction by the free edge of the cast. The swelling of the fingers or toes is indicative of increased pressure within the whole cast.
- Ease open the cut in the cast about $\frac{1}{4}$ to $\frac{1}{2}$ inch (0·6 to 1·25 cm).
- *Divide all padding including any wound dressings to expose the underlying skin.* Wound dressings must be cut as a blood-soaked gauze dressing dries rock hard and may itself form a constricting ring.
- *Check that bare skin is exposed throughout the whole length of the cut in the cast.* This is particularly important over the front of the ankle.
- Cut and place a strip of orthopaedic felt along the whole length of the opening in the cast. This will prevent herniation of the skin.
- Apply a crepe bandage around the cast.
- *Elevate the limb and encourage active movement of the toes or fingers.*

When impairment of circulation is due to an increase in pressure within a fascial compartment, the treatment is operative decompression of that compartment.

WEDGING A PLASTER CAST

The aim when reducing a fracture is to reduce overlap and to obtain correct apposition and alignment of the fragments without rotation at the fracture site. It is difficult to maintain reduction during the application of a plaster cast. Post-reduction radiographs may show that although length and apposition have been satisfactorily obtained and rotation corrected, angulation at the fracture site is present. This can be corrected by wedging the plaster cast.

Charnley (1970) states that wedging of plaster casts should be regarded as an unfortunate necessity rather than a procedure of choice.

A wedge may be of the opening or closing type. In practice an opening wedge is preferable (Watson Jones, 1932). Charnley (1970) states that he has the impression that there is a higher incidence of delayed union when an opening wedge is used. He advises that wedging should be completed within the first 2 to 3 days after the application of the first plaster cast. If however wedging is delayed until the fracture is 'sticky', distraction of the fracture and delayed union are less likely to occur. *Only wedge a padded plaster cast.*

HOW TO WEDGE A PLASTER CAST (Fig. 14.4)
- Study the antero-posterior and lateral radiographs to determine in which direction angulation has occurred.
- Identify the level of the fracture. This can be done by comparing the radiographs with the cast, or more accurately by taking a radiograph after attaching a radio-opaque marker to the cast.

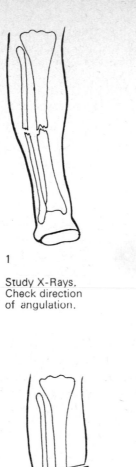

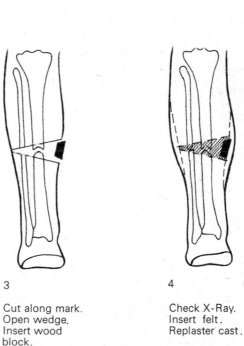

1
Study X-Rays.
Check direction
of angulation.

2
Identify level and
site of hinge.
Mark cast.

3
Cut along mark.
Open wedge.
Insert wood
block.

4
Check X-Ray.
Insert felt.
Replaster cast.

Figure 14.4   Wedging a plaster cast. Note: In the above diagrams, angulation is shown
on the antero-posterior X-ray only. If angulation is present on both the antero-posterior
and the lateral X-rays, the apex of the wedge will be antero-medial lateral or postero-
medial lateral, and the hinge must therefore be left at that site.

● Make a circumferential mark on the cast at the level of the fracture.
● Determine where on this mark the hinge of the wedge is to be located. The hinge is situated over the apex of the angulation when an opening wedge is proposed.
● Cut round the mark with an electric plaster saw, leaving 2 inches (2·5 cm) or one quarter of the circumference uncut, the site of the hinge.
● Slowly apply a corrective force to reduce the angulation, thus opening the wedge, the cast hinging on the uncut portion.
● Insert a wooden block to keep the wedge open. Temporarily secure the block with zinc oxide strapping.
● Take radiographs to determine whether adequate correction has been obtained. If not, open or close the wedge as required.
● If correction has been obtained, cut and insert a strip of orthopaedic felt the size of the wedge, *leaving the wooden block in place.*
● Apply plaster bandages around the cast.
● *Change the plaster cast—*
    1. If pain persists for more than 1 to 2 hours after wedging.
    2. *Routinely two weeks after wedging.* Any plaster cast can only be wedged once. If more correction is required, a new cast must be applied.

Complications of wedging of plaster casts

1. Embarrassment of the circulation in the limb.
2. Pressure sores.
3. Complete loss of the reduction.

REFERENCES

CHARNLEY, J. (1970) *The Closed Treatment of Common Fractures,* 3rd ed., p. 231. Edinburgh and London: Churchill Livingstone.
ENGLISH, M. (1957) *Plaster-of-Paris Technique.* Edinburgh: E. & S. Livingstone.
POWELL, M. (1968) *Orthopaedic Nursing,* 6th ed. Edinburgh and London: E. & S. Livingstone.
SMITH AND NEPHEW LTD. (1965) *Gypsona Technique,* 14th ed. Welwyn Garden City, Herts.
WATSON-JONES, R. (1932) The treatment of fractures of the shafts of the tibia and fibula. *Journal of Bone and Joint Surgery,* **14,** 591.

15. Tourniquets

In many orthopaedic operations on the upper or lower limbs such as nerve or tendon repair, a bloodless field is important. The recognition of tissues is easier, and trauma to tissues by repeated swabbing is eliminated.

A tourniquet has two functions, to arrest haemorrhage and to provide a bloodless field. Although only the provision of a bloodless field is considered here, much of what follows is applicable to the first function.

To provide a bloodless field, blood must be removed and prevented from re-entering a limb. Elevation for 5 minutes decreases the volume of blood in a limb as gravity increases the venous drainage. Reflex arteriolar constriction also occurs. More complete exsanguination of a limb is obtained by actively squeezing blood out of the limb. This is commonly achieved by using an Esmarch bandage (see below). To maintain a bloodless field the arterial supply must be obliterated. This is achieved by pressure from an encircling tightly applied rubber band or pneumatic cuff.

DANGERS OF A TOURNIQUET

Tourniquets are dangerous. The incorrect use of a tourniquet may cause damage to skin, muscles, blood vessels, nerves and other tissues. This damage may be caused by direct pressure on the tissues beneath the tourniquet itself, or by congestion or ischaemia of the tissues distal to the tourniquet. It may be so severe that amputation of the limb has to be performed (Watson-Jones, 1952).

The dangers from using a tourniquet result from—

1. **Incorrect placing of the tourniquet.** The tourniquet must be placed where the nerves and blood vessels are protected by muscle bulk, and where these structures are not likely to be compressed against bone. The correct site in the upper limb is around the arm and in the lower limb, around the upper thigh. The practice of placing a tourniquet around the calf should be discontinued.
2. **Failure to protect the skin.** The skin must be protected by wrapping a few layers of orthopaedic wool around the limb at the site of application of the tourniquet. Failure to do this may result in pinching and subsequent blistering of the skin.

181

3. **Excessive tourniquet pressure.** To maintain a bloodless field the pressure exerted by a tourniquet must exceed the systolic blood pressure. The subcutaneous fatty tissue and the muscles resist compression. The pressure required therefore depends upon the site of application of the tourniquet, the size of the limb and the level of the patient's systolic blood pressure. A higher pressure is required for adults, the lower limb and fat limbs, and a lower pressure for children, the upper limb and thin limbs. The pressures generally used are indicated below. *They will have to be modified for the individual patient.*

	ADULT	CHILD
UPPER LIMB (mm of Hg)	250	150
LOWER LIMB (mm of Hg)	500	250

4. **Excessive tourniquet time.** When a tourniquet is used, the tissues beneath and distal to the tourniquet are rendered ischaemic. Changes occur in the pH, pO_2, and pCO_2 values of these tissues, the extent of these changes (see below) being dependent upon the length of time the tourniquet is in place (Wilgis, 1971).

TOURNIQUET TIME	MEAN pH	MEAN pO_2 in mm	MEAN pCO_2 in mm
Before inflation	7·40	45	38
½ hour	7·31	24	50
1 hour	7·19	20	62
1½ hours	7·04	10	85
2 hours	6·90	4	104

Wilgis also found that after removal of the tourniquet, the venous and arterial pO_2 values at each interval are equal initially, but return to normal, taking 3–5 minutes after a tourniquet time of ½ hour, 5–10 minutes after 1 hour, 10–15 minutes after 1½ hours, and longer than 15 minutes after 2 hours, thus suggesting that during these intervals, oxygen diffusion across the capillary bed is minimal or absent due to shunting.

Striated muscle rendered ischaemic for two hours shows evidence of cell damage (Solonen and Hjelt, 1968). Below pH 7·2, the clotting time (in dogs) is increased (Rutherford *et al.*, 1966), and at a venous pO_2 of 10 mm, capillary permeability to fluid and protein increases (Webb, 1965).

These observations show that to minimise the potentially

harmful physiological changes which may occur with the use of a tourniquet, the length of time during which a tourniquet is used must be minimal. Time therefore must not be wasted. This can be achieved by careful pre-operative planning of the operation to avoid wasteful movements and by delaying the application of the tourniquet until all the necessary instruments are ready, the surgeon is scrubbed, gowned and ready to cleanse the skin, the patient is on the operating table and the operating light has been adjusted.

The time at which the tourniquet is applied is written down on a large board which is easily seen by all the operating room staff. The maximum length of time during which the limb may be kept ischaemic varies. Children and young adults appear to tolerate ischaemia better than the elderly. *One hour is the maximum length of time* generally accepted with an additional 30 minutes added if absolutely necessary. When an operation is likely to take longer, the tourniquet must be released to allow re-oxygenation of the tissues. Before releasing the tourniquet, moist packs are placed over the operative site and the limb is elevated to control bleeding. The longer the tourniquet has been in place, the longer must be the time allowed to elapse before the tourniquet is re-applied. After a tourniquet time of 1 hour allow 10 minutes, and after $1\frac{1}{2}$ hours allow 15 minutes.

To reduce the period of ischaemia, some surgeons release the tourniquet before suturing the skin. Others close the wound and apply a firm, well-padded dressing before releasing the tourniquet. The method practised will depend upon a number of factors which include the length of time the operative field may have been ischaemic, the possibility that large blood vessels may have been damaged and the ease with which any further procedures may be carried out without a bloodless field. However, it is generally agreed that the tourniquet must be released before the end of the operation when nerve suture or skin grafting is to be carried out. This is to avoid the formation of a haematoma between the nerve ends or under the skin graft.

5. **Failure to recognise injury to a major blood vessel** during the operation. Patrick (1963) described four cases of injury to the popliteal artery which occurred during operations for the removal of menisci. None of the injuries was recognised at the time of operation.

6. **Omitting to remove the tourniquet at the end of the operation.**

7. **Using a tourniquet when there are definite contra-indications to its use.**

CONTRAINDICATIONS TO THE USE OF A TOURNIQUET

1. *Peripheral arterial disease.*
2. *Sickle-cell disease.* Under anoxic conditions the red blood corpuscles sickle, blood viscosity increases, vessels become blocked and a severe episode of thrombosis and haemolysis may occur, particularly on release of the tourniquet. *Test all patients who are at risk* for the presence of Haemoglobin-S prior to the use of a tourniquet.
3. *Severe infections.* To avoid dissemination of the infection an exsanguinating tourniquet must not be used. Reduction of the volume of blood in the limb is obtained by elevation of the limb for 5 minutes.
4. *When proven or suspected deep vein thrombosis is present* an exsanguinating tourniquet must not be used. Austin (1963) reported two cases in which massive fatal pulmonary embolism was precipitated by exsanguination with an Esmarch bandage in the presence of silent deep vein thrombosis. Both patients had sustained fractures around the ankle, initially treated by manipulation and immobilisation in a plaster cast, which 7 to 9 days later required internal fixation.
5. *Severe crushing injuries.* In these cases the circulation is often precarious.

POST-TOURNIQUET SYNDROME

Following the release of a tourniquet there is reactive hyperaemia and congestion of the previously ischaemic tissues. Bruner (1951) stated that untoward tissue reactions were not noted when the duration of ischaemia was 20 to 30 minutes. Bunnell (1956) stated that one hour is safe but two hours gives some reaction. Certainly the longer the period of ischaemia and the older the patient the more likely it is that untoward tissue reactions will occur. These reactions are manifest in the hand (Bruner, 1951) by:

1. Puffiness of the hand and fingers, evidenced by a smoothing out of the normal skin creases.
2. Stiffness of the hand and finger joints to a degree not otherwise explained.
3. Colour changes in the hand which is pale in the horizontal position, more so when elevated and congested in the dependent position.
4. Subjective sensations of numbness in the affected hand without true anaesthesia.

5. Objective evidence of weakness in the muscles of the forearm without real paralysis.

He stated that these findings could be seen when the operative trauma and post-operative immobilisation of the hand were inadequate to explain these phenomena and where haematoma formation and infection were absent.

Swelling and stiffness of the hand and fingers after operation must be prevented, as the stiffness can become permanent due to fibrosis of the periarticular structures.

PREVENTION OF THE POST-TOURNIQUET SYNDROME

To decrease the degree of congestion of the tissues and to minimise haematoma formation at the operative site:

- **Select the correct operation for each patient.** As the tissues of elderly patients are less tolerant of ischaemia, swelling and stiffness are more likely to occur after operation. To carry out a lengthy operation may result therefore in a decrease rather than an increase in function.
- **Avoid wasting time.** It is imperative that the duration of tissue ischaemia is kept to a minimum. As already stated this is achieved by:
  Careful pre-operative planning of the operation to avoid wasteful movements.
  Delaying the application of the tourniquet until all necessary instruments are ready, the surgeon is scrubbed, gowned and ready to cleanse the skin, the patient is on the operating table and the operating lights are adjusted.
- **Do not extend the tourniquet time unnecessarily.** It is better to suture tendons after the tourniquet has been released rather than to prolong the duration of tissue ischaemia. Nerves must always be sutured and skin grafts applied after release of the tourniquet to avoid the formation of a haematoma between the nerve ends or under the skin graft.
- **Ensure good haemostasis.** If the tourniquet is released before the wound is closed, capillary haemorrhage is controlled by local pressure with saline compresses for 5 to 10 minutes, after which the larger vessels are clamped and ligated. If the wound is closed, a bulky dressing under moderate compression by a crepe bandage must be applied before the tourniquet is released.
- **Elevate the limb after the operation.**
- **Encourage the patient to perform active movements** of the pertinent part.

TOURNIQUET PARALYSIS SYNDROME

Tourniquet paralysis may result from excessive pressure, passive congestion of the part with haemorrhagic infiltration of the nerves when tourniquet pressure is too low, keeping the tourniquet on too long, the application of the tourniquet without consideration of the local anatomy (Smith, 1963), or applying a tourniquet on a very thin limb.

Characteristics of the tourniquet paralysis syndrome
(Moldaver, 1954)

Distal to the site of application of the tourniquet there are disturbances in the function of one or all of the nerves.

1. Motor paralysis with hypotonia or atonia but without appreciable atrophy.
2. Evidence of sensory dissociation. Touch, pressure, vibration and position sense usually are absent. The appreciation of pain is never lost and hyperalgesia is usually present. In severe cases the fast pain fibres may be affected, resulting in delay in the recognition of painful stimuli. The recognition of heat and cold is usually not affected. The patients do not complain of paraesthesia.
3. The sympathetic fibres are not affected.
4. The colour and temperature of the skin are normal.
5. All peripheral pulses are present.

Electrical studies of nerve conduction reveal a block to conduction, well localised to the site of application of the tourniquet. There is no response to stimulation of the motor nerves above the block, but stimulation below the block gives a good response. These studies show that tourniquet paralysis is caused by direct local mechanical pressure and not by generalised ischaemia of the limb.

When a tourniquet paralysis is complete, recovery may take up to three months, or longer.

ADVANTAGES AND DISADVANTAGES OF DIFFERENT TYPES OF TOUNIQUETS

Automatic pneumatic touniquet

1. An automatic pneumatic tourniquet can be fabricated from a blood pressure cuff attached by rubber tubing to a gas cylinder fitted with a pressure reducing valve and a manometer. The pressure in the cuff is furnished and maintained by gas from the cylinder. It is difficult however to pre-set the pressure accurately to the desired level.
2. The Kidde Automatic Tourniquet* which can be clamped to an infusion stand, utilizes a non-toxic, non-inflammable gas contained in a transparent gas reservoir. This permits a visual check

* See Appendix.

of the gas supply at any time during the use of the tourniquet. Rapid inflation of the cuff is possible. The pressure, regulated by a control knob which can be pre-set to the desired level, is maintained constant until changed by the control knob or by moving the inflate/deflate switch. The pneumatic cuffs are available in various sizes for use on children and upper and lower limbs.

The advantages of this type of tourniquet are that the pressure in the cuff is known, a continuous supply of gas from the cylinder or reservoir automatically compensates for any leaks in the system and as a gas reservoir is used, the patient is less likely to be moved from the operating table with the tourniquet in place.

Non-automatic pneumatic tourniquet

This consists of a pneumatic cuff, a hand-operated pump and a pressure gauge. The pressure in the cuff is known but there is no automatic compensation for leaks in the system and a regular check must be kept on the pressure in the cuff. In addition the hand-pump is small and it is easy to return the patient to the ward without removing the tourniquet.

Esmarch bandage

The Esmarch bandage (Esmarch, 1873) is a 3 inch (7·6 cm) wide and 6 yard (5·5 m) long india-rubber band, often with two tapes attached at one end. Although mainly used to exsanguinate a limb, it can be used as a tourniquet. Its use as a tourniquet is dangerous because the pressure exerted on the limb is unknown. Each turn adds to the pressure and hence to the risk of tourniquet paralysis. For this reason it must not be used on the upper limb. Its use on the lower limb is confined to the upper third of the thigh where the greater muscle bulk affords some protection to the underlying blood vessels and nerves.

HOW TO APPLY AN ESMARCH BANDAGE FOR EXSANGUINATION
An assistant is necessary.
- Elevate the limb.
- Wrap the Esmarch bandage around the limb, starting at the hand or foot and working proximally. The extreme tips of the fingers and toes and the heel can be left free.
- Fully stretch each turn of the bandage before applying it to the limb.
- Overlap each turn of the bandage by ½ inch (1·25 cm).

HOW TO APPLY AN ESMARCH TOURNIQUET

- Apply an Esmarch bandage as above.
- At the upper thigh wrap the Esmarch bandage over padding 4 to 5 times, all the turns except the first one being applied without stretching the bandage.
- Slip the remaining roll of the bandage under the last turn so that it lies in the line of the femoral artery.
- Tie the two end tapes to the table to guard against the patient leaving the theatre with the tourniquet still applied.
- Beginning at the toes remove the bandage.

HOW TO APPLY A PNEUMATIC TOURNIQUET

An assistant is necessary.

- Apply a few layers of orthopaedic wool, or a towel, around the limb at the tourniquet site.
- Choose the correct size of pneumatic cuff (upper limb, lower limb or paediatric).
- Express all air from the pneumatic cuff.
- Snugly wrap the pneumatic cuff around the limb on top of the padding.
- Ensure that the connecting tube lies on the outer aspect of the limb, and points proximally.
- Reinforce the Velcro, or other type of fastening of the pneumatic cuff, with zinc oxide strapping or a cotton bandage.
- Elevate the limb for 5 minutes, or—
- Exsanguinate the limb by applying an Esmarch bandage as described above, stopping the bandage 1 to 2 inches (2·5 to 5·0 cm) below the pneumatic cuff. If the Esmarch bandage is applied up to the level of the cuff, the cuff may slip distally at the time of inflation, or the pressure in the cuff may be so lowered on removal of the Esmarch bandage that bleeding may occur during the operation.
- Raise the pressure in the cuff rapidly to the predetermined level (see above) to prevent filling of the superficial veins before the arterial blood flow has been occluded.
- Note the time and write it down on a board.
- Remove the Esmarch bandage.

WHEN A TOURNIQUET IS USED:

- Use a colourless skin preparation solution especially for the toes and fingers. The state of the circulation in the toes or fingers will be determined more easily after the operation.
- Do not allow the skin preparation solution to collect under the edge of the tourniquet. Skin irritation or burning may result.
- If the pressure of the tourniquet should fall during the operation, remove the tourniquet completely to relieve congestion before reapplying it.
- Do not allow the tissues exposed at the operative site to become dry. Regularly apply cold saline compresses.
- Avoid the use of hot spot-lights which will accelerate the drying of the tissues.

● *At the end of the operation remove the tourniquet. This is the responsibility of the surgeon. Note the time at which the tourniquet is removed.*

● *At the end of the operation check that the circulation in the limb is satisfactory*—peripheral pulses and/or capillary circulation.

REFERENCES

AUSTIN, M. (1963) The Esmarch bandage and pulmonary embolism. *Journal of Bone and Joint Surgery,* **45-B**, 384.

BRUNER, J. M. (1951) Safety factors in the use of the pneumatic tourniquet for haemostasis in surgery of the hand. *Journal of Bone and Joint Surgery,* **33-A**, 221.

BUNNELL, S. (1956) *Surgery of the Hand,* 3rd ed., p. 90. Philadelphia: Lippincott.

ESMARCH, F. VON (1873) Ueber Kunstliche Blutleere bei Operationen. Sammlung Klinischer Vortrage in Verbindung mit Deutschen Klinikern. *Chirurgie,* **19**, No. 58, 373.

MOLDAVER, J. (1954) Tourniquet paralysis syndrome. *American Medical Association Archives of Surgery,* **68**, 136.

PATRICK, J. (1963) Aneurysm of the popliteal vessels after Meniscectomy. *Journal of Bone and Joint Surgery,* **45-B**, 570.

RUTHERFORD, R. B., WEST, R. L. and HARDAWAY, R. M. (1966) Coagulation changes during experimental haemorrhagic shock. *Annals of Surgery,* **164**, 203.

SMITH, H. (1963) Surgical Technique, Chapter 2, p. 22. *Campbell's Operative Othopaedics,* Volume Ij 4th ed. Edited by A. H. Crenshaw. St. Louis: C. V. Mosby Co.

SOLONEN, K. A. and HJELT, L. (1968) Morphological changes in striated muscle during ischaemia. *Acta Orthopaedica Scandinavica,* **39**, 13.

WATSON-JONES, R. (1952) *Fractures and Joint Injuries,* Vol. I, 4th ed., p. 121. Edinburgh: E. & S. Livingstone.

WEBB, W. R. (1965) Pulmonary physiology in surgery. Symposium on biologic foundations of surgery. *Surgical Clinics of North America,* **45**, 267.

WILGIS, E. F. S. (1971) Observations on the effects of tourniquet ischaemia. *Journal of Bone and Joint Surgery,* **53-A**, 1343.

16. Plastazote

There are a number of plastic materials used for orthopaedic appliances and splints. Plastazote (Smith & Nephew Ltd.)* is a foamed polyethylene of closed-cell construction, cross-linked to ensure extreme lightness and to improve its resistance to the temperature required for moulding. It is non-toxic, is unaffected by all common acids, alkalis and solvents, and is resistant to hot water and detergents. It is inflammable, but does not burn as readily as lint or cotton wool. Patients wearing Plastazote splints must avoid contact with naked flames or electric hot-plates as combustion can occur under such circumstances. When heated to 140° C, sheets of Plastazote will bond together and can be moulded. Due to its closed-cell structure, Plastazote is resilient, buoyant and will not absorb water. This makes it an ideal medium for supports worn in hydrotherapy pools.

APPLICATION OF PLASTAZOTE

Plastazote has a wide range of usage in the orthopaedic management of many conditions, and it is particularly useful in the construction of temporary supports, as the support can be made and finished within a few minutes. It has been used for the construction of cervical collars, spinal jackets, temporary insoles or permanent insoles where trophic ulceration is present, upper and lower limb splints, sandals and cradles for children suffering from fragilitas ossium. Because of its non-chafing and resilient properties, it is also used for the lining of plaster beds and amputation sockets. It is also very useful for making negative casts prior to the manufacture of block leather and plastic supports.

The method of making some of these appliances is described below. First, however, a description of the requisite equipment and some general points about the handling of Plastazote will be given.

> EQUIPMENT REQUIRED
> - A hot-air oven. The temperature must be thermostatically controlled at 140°C (range 135 to 145°C).
> - A sharp knife or scissors.
> - A tape measure.

* See Appendix.

- Sheets of Plastazote of varying thickness, and sheets of solid polyethylene.
- French chalk.
- A fine emery grinding wheel or No. 1 glasspaper for smoothing off the edges of the appliance.
- Retaining straps and fastenings.

General points about using Plastazote

1. Plastazote requires to be heated for 5 minutes in a hot-air oven at 140°C, after which time it can be moulded easily, and is auto-adhesive. As a result of this auto-adhesive property, sheets of Plastazote can be reinforced by placing strips of solid low-density polyethylene between them before heating. When this is done, 6 minutes are required in the oven. The temperature of the Plastazote after its removal from the oven must be checked carefully. This is very important when solid strips of polyethylene have been inserted for reinforcement because they retain heat longer than Plastazote. In addition great care must be taken to ensure that solid polyethylene does not project beyond the Plastazote sheets.
2. Plastazote can be moulded for 3 to 4 minutes after its removal from the oven. When it is laminated with strips of solid poly-ethylene, this time is extended slightly.
3. Trimming must not be done until the Plastazote is thoroughly cool.
4. Plastazote expands when heated.
5. To avoid the Plastazote sticking to the shelves in the oven, either the easy release paper which is supplied with the Plastazote, or French chalk must be used.
6. As sweating occurs under Plastazote appliances, they should be perforated.

HOW TO MAKE VARIOUS APPLIANCES

CERVICAL COLLAR
- Cut a sheet of $\frac{1}{2}$ inch (1·25 cm) Plastazote as shown in Figure 16.1.

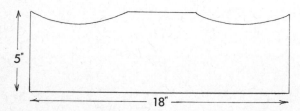

Figure 16.1   Shape of Plastazote for a cervical collar.

- Place the Plastazote in the oven and heat it for 5 minutes.
- Sit the patient beside the oven.
- Remove the Plastazote from the oven and check its surface temperature.
- Stand behind the patient, and place the Plastazote shape with the centre of the shaped edge (Fig. 16.1) on the chin. Stretch it gently but firmly first on one side and then the other around the neck. Avoid excessive pressure over the larynx especially in men.
- After 3 minutes remove the collar from the neck.
- When the Plastazote is cool, trim and smooth the edges.
- Reapply the collar, and check that it fits correctly before applying a retaining strap.

A reinforced cervical collar may be made from two $\frac{1}{4}$ inch (0·62 cm) sheets of Plastazote with a strip of solid polyethylene, $1\frac{1}{2}$ inches by $2\frac{1}{2}$ inches (3·75 cm by 6·25 cm), inserted anteriorly to support the chin.

SPINAL SUPPORT
Reinforcement with strips of solid polyethylene is generally required.

- Measure the patient from the mid-point of the sternum to the symphysis pubis and the circumference of the thorax and the buttocks. These measurements give the overall size of the sheets of Plastazote required.
- Cut two sheets of $\frac{1}{4}$ inch (0·62 cm) thick Plastazote to the required size.
- Cut four or more strips of solid polyethylene $1\frac{1}{2}$ inches (3·75 cm) wide to the required length and lay them between the sheets of Plastazote where reinforcement is required, taking care that they do not project beyond the edges of the Plastazote.
- Place a third piece of $\frac{1}{4}$ inch (0·62 cm) thick Plastazote over the area of the reinforcing strips (Fig. 16.2), on the side which is going next to the patient's skin.

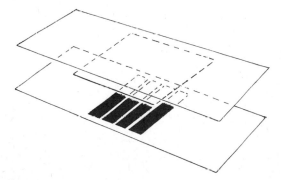

Figure 16.2 Plastazote spinal support. Note that the reinforcing strips of solid polyethylene are covered by a third piece of Plastazote sheet which is placed on the side next to the patient's skin.

- Heat in the oven for 5 minutes.
- Sit the patient beside the oven on a stool.
- Remove the Plastazote from the oven and check its surface temperature.
- Stretch the Plastazote pattern gently, firmly and quickly around the patient's trunk, from behind forwards, using the jacket clamp. A jacket clamp is a piece of wide, strong, elasticated webbing, fitted with webbing straps and wooden toggles.
- After 4 to 5 minutes remove the jacket from the patient, and when the Plastazote is cool, trim and smooth the edges.
- Reapply the jacket, check that it fits correctly and then apply three retaining straps.

FOREARM SPLINT

- In an 11 inches (27·5 cm) square sheet of ½ inch (1·25 cm) thick Plastazote cut a hole for the thumb. The diameter of this hole should be slightly less than the diameter of the metacarpo-phalangeal joint of the thumb. If a reinforced splint is required, ¼ inch (0·62 cm) sheets of Plastazote are used between which a piece of solid polyethylene is placed as shown in Figure 16.3.

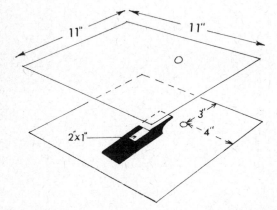

Figure 16.3 Lamination for reinforced forearm splint.

- Heat in the oven for 5 minutes.
- Remove the Plastazote from the oven and check its surface temperature.
- Place the patient's thumb through the hole, with the palm of the hand resting on the sheet of Plastazote, and mould the Plastazote round the hand and forearm on to the dorsum.
- After 3 to 4 minutes remove the splint, trim and smooth the edges.
- Apply three retaining straps.

FOOT SUPPORTS

- Cut three pieces measuring 12 inches by 4 inches (30 cm by 10 cm) from a sheet of 1 inch (2·5 cm) thick Plastazote.
- Put *two* of the above pieces in the oven to heat for 5 minutes.

- Place the third piece of Plastazote on the floor beside the patient's foot, as a cushion for the piece to be moulded.
- Remove one heated piece of Plastazote from the oven and dust French chalk over its *upper* surface and then place it on top of the unheated piece previously placed on the floor.
- Stand the patient with one foot on the pad for 2 to 3 minutes. While the patient is standing press the sides of the Plastazote up under the arches of the foot.
- Make a second support.
- After the Plastazote has cooled trim the insole down to fit into the patient's shoe, especially under the toes.

Vacuum-formed Plastazote footwear

Vacuum-formed Plastazote footwear is discussed in Chapter 11.

Appendix

Messrs.

George Salter Ltd.
    West Bromwich
    Staffordshire
    England.
	Suspension springs for a Thomas's splint.

Hangers Ltd.
    Limb Fitting Centre
    Rochampton
    Surrey
    England.
	Ortholene

Parke, Davis & Co.
    Pontypool
    Monmouthshire
    Wales.
	Ketalar (Ketamine Hydrochloride).

Performance Plastics Ltd.
    Melton Mowbray
    Leicestershire
    England.
	Perplas.

Pryor & Howard Ltd.
    Willow Lane
    Mitcham
    Surrey
    England.
	Fisk splint; brackets for attaching Böhler stirrup to Thomas's splint for suspension by springs.

Salt & Son Ltd.
    220 Corporation Street
    Birmingham
    England.
	Hartshill Lower Limb Appliances.

Seton Products Ltd.
    Tubiton House
    Medlock Street
    Oldham
    Lancashire
    England.
	Seton Skin Traction Kits: Tubi-grip.

Smith & Nephew Ltd.
  Bessemer Road
  Welwyn Garden City
  Hertfordshire
  England.

Elastoplast Skin Traction Kits.
  (Outside the British Common-
  wealth, all Elastoplast products
  are known under the name
  Tensoplast.) Plastazote and
  Technical Information Manual.

The Scholl Manufacturing Co.
  Ltd.
  182–204 St. John Street
  London
  England.

Ventfoam Skin Traction Bandage.

Victor Baldwin Ltd.
  Vansitard Estate
  Windsor
  Berkshire
  England.

Yampi, supplied in various colours.

Walter Kidde & Co. Inc.,
  Belleville
  New Jersey 07109
  U.S.A.

Kidde Automatic Tourniquet.

Zimmer Orthopaedic Ltd.
  176–178 Brompton Road
  London S.W.3
  England.

Orthotrac (in the U.S.A. it is called
  Orth-O-Trac): Zimmer Electric
  Plaster Saw.

Zimmer, U.S.A.
  727 North Detroit
  Warsaw
  Indiana 46580
  U.S.A.

Skin-Trac.

Index

Printed by T. & A. Constable Ltd, Edinburgh, Scotland